CON [barcode: T0091767]

JELLYFISH AGE BACKWARDS

NATURE'S SECRETS TO LONGEVITY

NICKLAS BRENDBORG

Translation by
Dr Elizabeth DeNoma
and Nicklas Brendborg

BACK BAY BOOKS
Little, Brown and Company
New York   Boston   London

Back Bay Books / Little, Brown and Company
Hachette Book Group
1290 Avenue of the Americas, New York, NY 10104
littlebrown.com

Originally published in the United Kingdom by Hodder Studio,
a division of Hodder & Stoughton: May 2022
Published in hardcover by Little, Brown and Company, January 2023.
First Back Bay trade paperback edition, February 2024

Back Bay Books is an imprint of Little, Brown and Company, a division of
Hachette Book Group, Inc.
The Back Bay Books name and logo are trademarks of Hachette Book Group, Inc.

The publisher is not responsible for websites (or their content)
that are not owned by the publisher.

The Hachette Speakers Bureau provides a wide range of authors for
speaking events. To find out more, go to hachettespeakersbureau.com or
email HachetteSpeakers@hbgusa.com.

Little, Brown and Company books may be purchased in bulk for business,
educational, or promotional use. For information, please contact your local
bookseller or the Hachette Book Group Special Markets Department
at special.markets@hbgusa.com.

ISBN 978-0-316-41458-6 (hc) / 978-0-316-41468-5 (pb)
LCCN is available at the Library of Congress.

10 9 8 7 6 5 4 3 2 1

CW

Printed in the United States of America

The Fountain of Youth

In 1493, an expedition of seventeen ships left the Spanish port town of Cádiz. After a stop in the Canary Islands, the expedition ventured out across the Atlantic. Destination: India. Maybe?

This convoy was the second Spanish voyage to America. The aim was to establish the first Spanish base in the New World, and to do so, the commander, Christopher Columbus, brought more than a thousand men with him. Among them was the young and ambitious Juan Ponce de León. When the expedition reached its destination – the tropical island of Hispaniola – Ponce de León settled down and eventually became a respected military commander and landowner.

At the time, the New World was a place of legends involving strange lands, alien peoples and, of course, massive wealth. One day, Ponce de León heard just such a story promising new land north of Hispaniola. He quickly assembled a crew and set out to investigate. Ponce de León's expedition ventured north along the Bahamas and then glimpsed a strange new place, which they named *La Florida* for the many flowers in the landscape.

The Spaniards were quick to explore the new land and at one point, they encountered a tribe of native peoples. During the meeting, the natives told the Spaniards about a mythical spring, which they called the 'Fountain of Youth': a spring whose water was healing and which could make even the oldest person young again. They insisted, however, that no one in their community could remember where it was. And no, no, they didn't just tell this story to make the Spaniards leave them alone. It was completely true.

In the following years, the Spanish expedition traversed the coast of Florida, searching every nook and cranny for this infamous source of immortality. The hopeful Spaniards plunged into every freshwater spring they found – pretty brave, considering Florida's alligator population. Of course, the Spaniards never found the mythical spring, and in turn, the Grim Reaper eventually found them all.

★ ★ ★

Alright, serious historians will probably tell you that the Fountain of Youth story is mostly a myth. Fortunately, I'm not a serious historian, so I'm allowed to start my book with a bit of a tall tale.

Truth be told, Ponce de León and his men were probably seeking the same kind of fortune as everyone else at the time: land and gold, probably slaves and undoubtedly also women. Nevertheless, tales of the quest for eternal life recur across every single civilisation we know. There are accounts of rejuvenating springs and immortalising elixirs in every historical culture, from Alexander the Great in ancient Greece, to the Crusaders, ancient India, ancient China, ancient Japan and everywhere in between.

In fact, one of the oldest pieces of literature *ever* is about just this very subject. The *Epic of Gilgamesh*, which dates back more than 4,000 years, tells the story of a king who leaves his people and travels to the end of the world in search of immortality. Contemporary civilisation is no exception. Though we've mostly moved on from magic springs and elixirs, we still long to uncover the secrets behind a long life. However, today, the main source of these stories is not legends and myths but scientific research. You'd think this would be unquestionable progress, but that hasn't always been the case. Science has had a few bumps on the road towards understanding ageing.

In the early twentieth century, some scientists believed that extracts from animal glands could be used to rejuvenate humans. One of these researchers, the surgeon Serge Voronoff, was convinced that consuming the animal extracts or doing infusions was not enough; no, you needed to transplant tissue directly on to people for the desired effect. After studying castrated men in Egypt, Voronoff concluded that testicles were the number one source of rejuvenation.

Naturally, he began grafting small pieces of monkey testicles on to his patients. The treatment was bizarre enough for ordinary people to avoid it like the plague. But the rich and famous *loved* it; they lined up in droves to try Voronoff's miraculous anti-ageing grafts. In fact, there was so much interest that Voronoff made a ton of money, and soon he started having difficulty obtaining enough monkey testicles. To secure his supply, he had to create an enclosure for the poor animals at the castle he'd bought, and hire a circus trainer to breed them.

Of course, Voronoff's patients didn't end up as anything but a historical joke. They and Voronoff grew old and frail, just like Ponce de León and his men. And just like we will – unless science can find a better solution than what's come before.

That's what this book is about – how to 'die young' as late as possible. In other words, about the nature and science of longevity and a healthy life. I promise you that you won't have to sew testicles to your thigh, or swim with flesh-eating reptiles. But nevertheless, it will be something of a journey.

Part I

NATURE'S WONDERS

Chapter 1

The Record Book of Longevity

Beneath the surface of the ice-blue Greenland Sea glides a huge shadow. The twenty-foot giant isn't in a hurry; its top speed is less than two miles per hour.

In Latin it's called *Somniosus microcephalus* – 'the sleepwalker with the tiny brain'. In English, it has a slightly more flattering name: the Greenland shark. As its Latin name suggests, this shark is neither fast nor particularly quick-witted – though despite this, you can find the remains of seals, reindeer and even polar bears in its stomach.

Our mysterious companion takes its time because time is something it has a lot of. When the United States was founded, it was already older than any human has ever been. When the *Titanic* sank, it was 281 years old. And now, it's just turned 390. Despite this, researchers estimate that it could have several more years to live.

This is not to say that the Greenland shark has no problems. Its eyes are infected with bioluminescent parasites that are slowly making it blind. And, despite its impressive size, the Greenland shark shares an enemy with all other inedible fish – Icelanders. You see, the flesh of a Greenland shark contains so much of a toxic substance called trimethylamine N-oxide that you get dizzy – 'shark-drunk' – from eating it. But, of course, the brave people of Iceland have found a way to do so anyway.

The Greenland shark is exactly the kind of animal that belongs at the top of some kind of list. And that *is* where we find it. With its impressive lifespan, the Greenland shark is the longest-lived vertebrate ever recorded. Being a vertebrate – an animal with a backbone – it is actually our distant relative. We might not look much alike, but the basic anatomy is recognisable: a heart, a liver, an intestinal system, two kidneys and a brain.

Of course, there is still quite some distance on the evolutionary tree between us and a giant fish. Humans are mammals, and that means we have certain fundamental characteristics that we don't share with the Greenland shark. In biology, the rule of thumb is that the closer an animal is to us in evolutionary terms, the more we can learn about ourselves from studying it. That means we can learn more from fish than from insects, but also that we can learn less from fish than we can from, for instance, birds and reptiles. Not to mention our closest relatives – other mammals.

Oddly enough, the Greenland shark shares its home with another lifespan record-holder that is a much closer relative of ours. If you're fortunate in the seas around Greenland, you might encounter the sixty-foot-long bowhead whale. While the surface characteristics of a bowhead whale don't resemble ours either, its inner wiring is much closer to humans than that of the Greenland shark. Whales have large brains, even for their size, four-chambered hearts like us, lungs and many other common characteristics.

We used to hunt these magnificent animals to use their blubber in oil lamps, but fortunately they are protected today. Only native peoples, such as the Iñupiat people of Alaska, are allowed to continue hunting them – at subsistence levels, as they have always done. Occasionally, after a successful hunt, the Iñupiat will visit local authorities to hand off old harpoon tips recovered from the whales' blubber. These harpoon tips stem from unsuccessful hunts in the 1800s. Together with molecular methods, they have been used to determine that bowhead whales can live more than 200 years. That's the longest lifespan recorded for a mammal.

Moving away from humans on the evolutionary tree can reveal some even more impressive lifespans. The best examples come from actual trees, for whom ageing doesn't really exist – at least, not in the way that we typically understand it. While our own risk of dying increases as we age, trees only get larger, stronger and hardier. That means trees have a *decreased* risk of dying each year they live. At least up to the point where they get so tall that they get knocked over in a storm. But dying in an accident has nothing to do with ageing.

This means that some trees are *really* old. One of the oldest single trees, Methuselah, is a 5,000-year-old bristlecone pine in a secret location somewhere in the White Mountains of California. At the time Methuselah sprouted from the soil, the pyramids were still being built in Egypt and the last mammoths roamed Wrangel Island in Siberia.

Yet even Methuselah is a spring chicken compared to the wooden record-holder. In the Utah Fishlake National Forest, roughly 350 miles northeast of Methuselah, is an American aspen named Pando. Pando (Latin for 'I spread') is not a single tree, but a kind of superorganism – a giant network of roots filling an area around one eighth the size of Central Park in New York.

Pando is the heaviest organism on the planet and sprouts more than 40,000 individual trees. Most of these trees live between 100 and 130 years, dying off in storms, fires and so on. But Pando continuously sprouts new trees, and the root network superorganism itself is more than 14,000 years old.

The Queen of Tonga

Obviously, I can't write a chapter on exceptionally long-lived organisms without mentioning turtles. One of the oldest turtles ever was the radiated tortoise Tu'i Malila, who lived with the royal family of the tropical island kingdom of Tonga. Tu'i Malila was given as a gift to the King of Tonga by the British explorer James Cook in 1777. When she died in 1965, as a very old lady, she had lived about 188 years. That's the age record for any turtle whose age we can verify with certainty. However, Tu'i Malila is about to be overtaken by the Seychelles giant tortoise, Jonathan, who lives on the tiny Atlantic island of Saint Helena. Jonathan was hatched around 1832 – before the invention of the postage stamp – and has lived through the reigns of seven British monarchs and the terms of thirty-nine US presidents. By the time you're reading this, Jonathan might be the new record-holder.

While some organisms can live significantly longer than us, others have different ageing trajectories altogether. That is, ageing happens to some organisms in a completely different way than it does to us.

As humans, we age exponentially; after puberty, our risk of dying doubles approximately every eight years. This happens as our physiology gradually declines, making us ever frailer. Our way of ageing is the most common one and we share it with most of the animals we're in daily contact with. However, it is by no means the only pattern of ageing in nature.

There's a particularly weird group of animals that reproduce only once, followed by immediate and rapid ageing. This is called semelparity, and if you like watching nature documentaries, you might recognise it from the life cycle of Pacific salmon.

Pacific salmon hatch in small streams, where the tiny salmon mature in relative safety. Later, they head out to sea, where they stay until eventually becoming sexually mature. At some point, it's time to make the next generation of Pacific salmon, but unfortunately the salmon only breed in the exact stream in which they hatched themselves. That means the poor fish must swim back inland – sometimes a distance of hundreds of miles – *against* the current and *uphill*. It still boggles my mind that any fish is actually able to make it *up* a waterfall. It's a wild journey.

Even more unfortunate for salmon is the fact that we are not the only animals aware of how tasty they are. When the salmon start migrating, every single local predator – bears, wolves, eagles, herons and so on – is patiently waiting, ready to feast. To give itself a shot, the Pacific salmon pumps its body full of stress hormones and completely stops eating. Every day and night becomes a tireless battle against Mother Nature herself. Most salmon don't make it, but the few who do go on to spawn the next generation in the very streams in which their own lives began.

Having achieved this feat, you might think the hardy salmon would have no problems returning to the sea. After all, this trip would be *downhill* and helped along by the current. But the salmon show no interest in even trying. Once they've spawned, they go into terminal decline, like plants withering in an instant. A few days after hiding their fertilised eggs in the sandy riverbed, the entire previous generation is dead.

This kind of bizarre and rather tragic life story is actually more widespread in nature than you might think. Here are some of my other favourite examples:

- Once female octopuses have laid their eggs, their mouths seal up, they stop eating, and they dedicate their entire selves to protecting the eggs. A few days after their eggs hatch, the mothers die.
- The males of the small mouse-like Australian marsupial *Antechinus stuartii* get so stressed, aggressive and sexually exhausted during the mating season that they die shortly after.
- Cicadas spend most of their lives (up to seventeen years) underground, coming to the surface only to lay eggs. Soon afterwards, they die.
- Mayflies don't live more than a day or two after hatching. In fact, there's a certain type of fly that doesn't have a mouth and only lives for about five minutes. Its only mission is to reproduce once.
- There are even some plants that display this pattern of ageing. American aloe, which is also known as century plant, can live for decades, but shortly after blooming for the first and only time, it withers and dies.

Conversely, there are also some animals that don't age at all – at least, not in the way we traditionally define ageing. One such example is the lobster. Just like trees, the king of the crustaceans doesn't get weaker or less fertile as time passes. Quite the contrary, actually – lobsters grow continuously throughout their lives and get stronger and stronger over time. Of course, this doesn't mean that they live forever. Nature is cruel, and eventually predators, competitors, diseases or accidents will do the job. If not, the biggest lobsters end up dying from physical problems due to their large size. Old age for a lobster, however, is not at all the gradual decline we know ourselves.

★ ★ ★

Nature also hosts organisms that have developed some truly peculiar tricks to prolong life. Some bacteria, for example, can go into a kind of dormant state. When stressed, the bacterium transforms itself into a compact structure resembling a seed. This structure, called an endospore, is resilient to anything nature might expose it to – even extreme heat and ultraviolet radiation. Inside the endospore, the processes normally required to sustain the bacterium are all paused. It's as if the bacterium isn't even alive anymore. However, the endospore can still sense its surroundings. When times get better, it can unpack itself and become a fully active bacterium again like nothing ever happened.

Exactly how long bacteria can spend in their dormant state is hard to say. Maybe there's not really a limit at all. It's routine practice for scientists to revive endospores that they have found which are over 10,000 years old. In fact, there are reports of endospores being awakened after millions of years of dormancy.

I think, however, that I would give the prize of 'greatest ageing trick' to the tiny jellyfish *Turritopsis*, the namesake of this book. To the untrained eye, *Turritopsis* seems kind of dull. It's a tiny jellyfish roughly the size of a fingernail that spends its life drifting around eating plankton.

But treat it right and *Turritopsis* might reveal its secret.

If the tiny jellyfish is stressed – for example, by hunger or sudden temperature changes in the water – something strange happens: it reverts from its adult form to something called the polyp stage. This is akin to a butterfly turning back into a caterpillar, or to you having a stressful day at work and deciding to revert to being a kindergartner again.

When *Turritopsis* returns to its polyp stage, it is in fact ageing backwards. Afterwards, it can grow up anew with no physiological recollection of having been older. To make this Benjamin

Button-esque trick even more impressive, research suggests that *Turritopsis* can repeat its rejuvenation again and again. Obviously, being a tiny jellyfish in a huge ocean means that *Turritopsis* doesn't live forever in the wild. Eventually, something will eat it. However, it's quite possible that it *could* live forever in the safety of a laboratory. *Turritopsis* may well be an example of the holy grail of ageing research – biological immortality.

As it is with all good ideas, though, odds are someone else had it too. While *Turritopsis* is my favourite example of backwards ageing, nature actually has other examples too, including another 'immortal' jellyfish, *Hydra,* and a primitive flatworm called *Planaria.* When there is plenty of food, *Planaria,* like *Turritopsis,* lives an unimpressive life. But if its food disappears, it reveals a special trick. A starved *Planaria* will eat itself, starting with the least important parts, and it doesn't stop until nothing but the nervous system is left. This buys the flatworm time in the hope that conditions improve. When *Planaria* senses that better times are ahead, it can then rebuild itself and begin its life anew. While other worms of a similar age die, the rejuvenated *Planaria* will swim around, still full of youthful energy. In fact, the *Planaria* flatworm is so good at regenerating itself that you can cut it in half and – instead of ending up with two halves of a dead flatworm, you end up with two living worms.

Imagine if we could one day learn how these animals work their magic.

★ ★ ★

Bowhead whales live a long time. So do twenty-foot Greenland sharks and large tortoises. Do you detect a pattern? How about if I told you the average mouse has to be lucky to live for two years – even in the protection of captivity?

The secret these long-lived animals share is their size. In general, large animals live longer than small ones. Whales, elephants and humans are long-lived. Most rodents are not.

The evolutionary reason is probably that size protects against predators. When the risk of becoming someone else's dinner is smaller, there can be an evolutionary pay-off from a slow life course. That is, a life course characterised by maturing slowly, having few offspring that are nurtured for long periods of time and investing in the upkeep of the body. On the other hand, if a species is constantly in danger, it doesn't make much sense to live for the future. Instead, such a species should mature as quickly as possible, disregard the future for the present and get a ton of offspring in the hope that fate will be kind to at least some of them.

One example that brilliantly illustrates this trade-off is the opossum. Biologist Steven Austad was studying these small marsupials in the Venezuelan rainforest, when he began to wonder why they seemed to age so rapidly. If Austad caught the same opossum twice, there would be visible physical differences, even after just a few months.

Photos of the rainforest might make it look like paradise, but in reality it is more like a tropical nightmare for its inhabitants. Danger lurks behind every tree trunk and the life course of the resident opossums reflects that. The opossums have evolved to focus less on bodily upkeep and instead on the mission of reproducing before something eats them. Conversely, Austad also managed to find a population of opossums living in something that is akin to opossum paradise. On Sapelo Island, off the coast of Georgia in the United States, there are no predators, and the local opossums spend their days lounging in the sun, carefree. This population of opossums has lived in relative protection for thousands of years. And as a result, they have evolved longer lifespans than their mainland cousins – when the likelihood of surviving is higher, there's a bigger pay-off for focusing on bodily upkeep.

That a relatively safe life allows the evolution of a longer lifespan could also explain our own special status: even though humans are large mammals, we live longer than you'd expect from our size alone. The reason is probably that we're at the pinnacle of the food chain. Most animals are smart enough to avoid us and you can imagine the ones that weren't so inclined learned the hard way back in the Stone Age.

Similarly, this hypothesis also explains some of the exceptions to the rule about size and lifespan. Most of the small animals that have managed to buck the trend share a similar adaptation which helps when evading predators: they can fly. For instance, birds live longer than mammals of the same size. And the only flying mammals, bats, live three-and-a-half times longer than other mammals of a similar size.

★ ★ ★

Now that I have convinced you that large animals live longer than small ones, which dog breed do you think lives the longest: a Great Dane or a chihuahua? If you're a dog lover with a preference for larger breeds, you might know that one of the tragedies of this love story is that large dogs don't live very long. A Great Dane will typically live for around eight years, while small dogs, such as chihuahuas, Jack Russells and Lhasa Apsos, can live more than twice that long. The reason is that while large animal species live longer than small animal species, the opposite is true *within* each species. That is, small individuals live longer than large individuals. Ponies live longer than horses, for instance, while the species lifespan record-holder for mice is held by something called the Ames dwarf mouse.

In the same way, female mammals almost always live longer than males of the same species. This rule holds whether you're looking at lions, deer, prairie dogs, chimpanzees, gorillas or humans. But why? One clue is that female mammals are almost always smaller than their male counterparts. Among humans, men's bodies are fifteen to twenty per cent larger, and on average women live a few years longer. In the few species of mammal where males and females are equally sized, like hyenas, males and females have roughly equal lifespans.

★ ★ ★

We've yet to meet the animal that life-extension researchers hold dearest of all.

Our anti-ageing all-star originates in East Africa, but is nowhere to be seen in the vast savannah landscape. Dig a few inches underground, though, and this tiny animal can be found scampering away through the miles-long tunnels it's constructed.

The naked mole-rat, as this creature is called, is not a favourite among scientists due to its looks. Imagine the rat from your worst nightmares, and then keep going. Its skin is bald, pink and wrinkled. Scattered long hairs protrude from its body. Its front teeth, used for digging, are located *outside* the mouth. And its barely functional eyes are nothing but tiny black dots.

Despite its looks, though, the naked mole-rat has plenty of friends. The creature's East African tunnel kingdoms are built and maintained by colonies of 20 to 300 members who patrol them in search of enemies and food.

When off-duty, colony members reside at the headquarters, where there are rooms for food storage, sleeping quarters and even toilets. The colony's headquarters is also the domain of the most special naked mole-rat of all: the queen. You see, a colony of naked mole-rats does not work like a normal herd of mammals. Instead, the small rats are some of the only mammals that are *eusocial*, the type of social structure we more commonly associate with insects such as ants and bees. The queen is the only naked mole-rat to have cubs, while the rest of the colony consists of temporarily sterile workers and soldiers – except for a few males that the queen has selected as her boytoys.

Researchers of ageing find naked mole-rats so fascinating because they don't conform to the usual correlation between size and lifespan. An adult naked mole-rat weighs about thirty-five grams, which is not much heavier than a mouse. Despite this, naked mole-rats live well over thirty years, while the species record for mice is about four years.

To understand the importance of all this, imagine the following: you're a researcher who wants to study ageing. Where do you look for inspiration? An obvious option is to study long-lived animals – maybe you can learn some of their secrets.

You think to yourself: Animals that live a long time . . . whales? Those would be a little hard to keep in the laboratory. Elephants? Same problem. Birds in little cages? Animal torture (besides, they aren't even mammals). How about the naked mole-rat? Long-lived? Check. Can be kept in a laboratory? Check. A mammal like us? Check. So far, so good.

The next challenge you face is finding something to which you can compare your animal. The obvious choice is to use a short-lived relative. Then you can examine the differences between the two to see if you can explain their dissimilar lifespans. Here, again, it turns out that the naked mole-rat is a perfect choice. The two most-studied laboratory animals – mice and rats – happen to be closely related to the naked mole-rat while having very dissimilar lifespans. So this little creature is perfect for studying ageing.

Researchers around the world have beaten us to it and have been studying naked mole-rats for decades by now. These researchers report that it's almost impossible to tell the difference between young and old naked mole-rats. One might add that the threshold for looking young is pretty low for a naked mole-rat: you just have to be hairless and wrinkled. Nonetheless, it's an interesting observation. Not only do scientific tests *show* that naked mole-rats age slowly— we can also *see* it.

Naked mole-rat researchers also report that their animals are virtually immune to cancer, even when the researchers try to induce it artificially. Out of the thousands of mole-rats studied, only six tumours have ever been found. That's particularly remarkable in such a small animal. By comparison, signs of cancer can be found in seventy per cent of all laboratory mice after their deaths. And, in general, it is normal for twenty to fifty per cent of individuals to get cancer in any given species, including our own. In many developed countries, for example, cancer has overtaken cardiovascular diseases as the most prolific killer. And yet somehow, this small, obscure rodent from East Africa has found a way to tame the disease. A miraculous creature indeed, and one that has a central role to play in our unfolding story of ageing.

Chapter 2

Sun, Palm Trees and a Long Life

On a warm Thursday at around noon, a converted school bus rolls into the bus terminal in the Costa Rican town of Nicoya, the capital of the peninsula bearing the same name. I manage to confirm that this is my bus and I join the growing line of locals waiting to get on: young mothers, elderly couples, middle-aged women and laughing schoolchildren. We all get in place and soon the bus winds its way out through the concrete jungle of Nicoya and further into the lush Costa Rican countryside. Along the traffic-free road are small, colourful houses, and on the horizon a deep green landscape appears.

Inside the bus, the lone gringo quickly attracts attention. I have to disappoint: 'No hablo español'. However, that doesn't prevent a basic conversation from developing anyway. Through a combination of hand gestures, guidebook Spanish and a little Google Translate, we're able to communicate.

After a while, a woman turns to me cautiously and addresses me in broken English: 'Are you going to Hojancha?'

I am.

But why? Am I going hiking?

No, not really. 'I'm here to see the Blue Zone,' I explain.

The woman laughs and translates for a few of the others. Then she looks at me more seriously. 'It's true what they say.'

Half an hour later the bus rolls into the central square of the sleepy village of Hojancha. When I get off the bus, a local man shows me the best restaurant in town while thanking me several times for my visit. Then, while I'm enjoying my casado, everyday life in rural Costa Rica unfolds around me.

★ ★ ★

Pessimists might claim that we will never be able to win the fight against ageing or even to seriously prolong life. But that view is hard to share when you know about ageing in nature. Other animals, just as complex as us in their own right, can live for significantly longer than us, go long periods without ageing, or even age *backwards*. That makes it hard to believe there are fundamental biological limits anywhere close to our current lifespans. With some ingenuity, we have the ball at our feet.

But while inspiration from the natural world might one day help us combat ageing, it is not the only place to look for ideas. We can learn a lot from our fellow humans as well. We're obviously all very similar, but there are still differences in how well we age and how long we live. And this is where the Nicoya Peninsula comes into the picture. The mountainous Costa Rican region is a popular tourist destination due to its incredible scenery: pristine rainforest, beautiful sandy beaches and a warm, pleasant climate. But in addition, the Nicoya Peninsula is known thanks to its featured role in the book *The Blue Zones* by American journalist Dan Buettner. In the book, Buettner visits regions of the globe known as 'Blue Zones' where locals have a particularly high probability of attaining advanced ages.

Besides the Nicoya Peninsula, there are four other Blue Zones: the Barbagia region of Sardinia (Italy), the island of Ikaria (Greece), the prefecture of Okinawa (Japan) and the city of Loma Linda (California, USA). The inhabitants of all these places boast some pretty incredible lifespan statistics. Take, for instance, those born in the year 1900. Okinawan women born that year were over seven-and-a-half times more likely to become centenarians (reach 100 years old) than women from my native Denmark. And for men, the probability of becoming a centenarian was almost six times higher in Okinawa than in Denmark.

So the question is, what is it about these seemingly random areas of the globe that produces such long-lived inhabitants? Either there's something special about the people or there is something special about their lifestyles and surroundings.

At first glance, we might be tempted by a genetic explanation. It's noticeable that all five Blue Zones are somewhat isolated. Even today, many of the transport routes on Nicoya are small jungle trails or dirt roads, where your best bet for getting around is an ATV. This means that the inhabitants have been historically isolated and married locally. If favourable ageing genetics existed in Nicoya, they would have made the rounds for many generations. However, relatedness cannot be the sole explanation. Studies show that when locals move away from the Nicoya Peninsula, they don't live as long as those who have stayed.

Dan Buettner's attempt at an explanation revolves around the cultures of these regions: the tightness of families there, the food that's eaten, the active yet relaxed way of life, and the strong sense of meaning among the inhabitants.

Buettner might be right, but we don't have much time to find out. In the last decades, the long arm of globalisation has taken a firm grip on the Blue Zones. Today, the lifestyle of a person on the Nicoya Peninsula is converging with that of the rest of the world. There's lots of fast food, sedentary work, and most people use motorised transportation. In remote mountain villages, you can still find hints of the old way of life, but even here there are satellite dishes on the rooftops and cars in the driveways.

The Okinawa prefecture in Japan is a particularly good example of the deflation of the Blue Zones. Right up until the turn of the millennium, the people of Okinawa had the longest average life expectancy in all of Japan. That's saying something when the Japanese are already notoriously long-lived. However, since then, this Blue Zone has disappeared before our eyes. Today, Okinawans have one of the highest average BMIs among Japanese prefectures and eat the most KFC, while the island has dropped drastically in longevity rankings and is now among the lowest ranked prefectures in Japan.

By and large, the developments in Okinawa and the other Blue Zones are, of course, a form of progress. Globalisation might have brought obesity and health problems, but it has also ushered in access to modern medicine, clean drinking water and safety from the pain of starvation. Life on the Nicoya Peninsula is probably better today than it used to be. But the rapid economic development of the region makes it hard for us to understand what the secrets of the Blue Zones are. Or rather, what they were.

★ ★ ★

Critics of the Blue Zone concept argue that globalisation hasn't hurt these places at all. Perhaps they were never long-lived to begin with. You see, after the US introduced state-wide birth certificates, the number of very old people dropped sharply. That's not because birth certificates kill people. It turns out a lot of 'centenarians' were just innumerate people unaware of their actual age – or, if you adopt the harsher perspective, straight-up frauds. Critics argue that most of the Blue Zones could be seeing fraud of this kind, too. They reason that Sardinia, Okinawa and Ikaria are curious places for attaining a high age. They're remote and poor provinces, characterised by low education levels, relatively high crime rates, high alcohol consumption and high smoking rates.

Now, Blue Zone researchers are not naive and have obviously thought of this angle. They have worked hard to validate the actual ages of the people they study using official documents, interviews with family members and lots of cross-checking. However, it is hard to rule out fraud completely. Fraud has definitely been the cause of other 'longevity hotspots' in the past. And one thing is certain: lying about your age is one of the oldest forms of fraud there is. Myths, legends and even historical sources are littered with people who supposedly lived 200, 500 or even 1,000 years. This fact is important to keep in mind going forwards as we discuss studies of centenarians.

If we want to learn about human longevity, it might be safer to look at country-level data instead. In this case, our best bet is the list of average life expectancies around the world published by the World Health Organization. At the time of writing, this list is topped by Japan, followed by Switzerland, South Korea, Singapore and Spain. Positions change from year to year, but in general, the list is a *Who's Who* of the world's rich democracies. Besides that, it is noticeable that developed Asian countries do particularly well. While Japan, South Korea and Singapore are all rich countries, their inhabitants live even longer than might be expected from their wealth alone. The reason for this is currently unknown. One explanation could be healthy lifestyles. Asian countries tend to have healthier food cultures and lower obesity rates than Western countries. But on the other hand, they also tend to have higher smoking rates and higher levels of pollution. Another explanation could be extensive pension fraud. For instance, in 2010, Japanese authorities found that 230,000 of the people listed as centenarians were unaccounted for. Some of these people might have died long ago without being reported so that their relatives could keep receiving their pensions. But then again, there's nothing to suggest pension fraud should be more common in Asia than in the rest of the world. And besides, Asian immigrants and their descendants also live long lives in the United States. In fact, they are the longest-lived ethnicity in the country, living longer than Americans of European descent.

Zooming in on my own corner of the world, it is also noticeable that Southern European countries tend to out-perform their Northern neighbours. At the time of writing, Spain, Cyprus and Italy are numbers two, three and four in Europe. These countries have life expectancies around two years higher on average than some of the more poorly per-forming Northern European countries, such as Germany, the UK and – it saddens me to say – my native Denmark. The European Blue Zones, Ikaria and Sardinia, are both located in Southern Europe, and I think the rankings accurately reflect the stereotypes held by most Europeans. The 'Mediterranean diet' has long been touted as especially health-promoting, for instance.

So while it is no surprise that the inhabitants of rich coun-tries generally live longer than those of poor countries, it seems we should particularly look to East Asia and Southern Europe if we really want to learn about human longevity.

Chapter 3

Genes Are Overrated

When explaining our differences, the social sciences usually distinguish between heredity and environment – nature versus nurture. That is, our traits may be innate (something in our genes), or they may be learned (something that has been shaped by our experiences). For example, if you had been adopted by a purple-eyed family in Bulgaria as an infant, that wouldn't change your own eye colour. But it would mean that you would be speaking Bulgarian today, not English. That's because eye colour is genetically determined while language is environmentally determined.

Though this clear distinction works for a few traits, it is somewhat artificial. The vast majority of our traits are due to both genetics *and* environment. Take your personality. You have some natural inclinations – maybe you are a little temperamental or shy, for example. But it can get much better (or worse) depending on what kind of upbringing you had and what environment you find yourself in.

In the same way, we would expect our health and longevity to be affected by both genes and environment. If we want to learn about ageing and find ways to combat it, we should try to untangle the contribution of each.

The most commonly used method for studying genes versus environment is twin studies. Here, scientists take advantage of a gift from nature: the fact that identical twins have the same DNA. They are like genetic clones. You see, normally, after a sperm cell fertilises an egg, the fertilised egg will develop into a single person. However, sometimes, there can be a split during early cellular divisions. When this happens, the fertilised egg ends up becoming *two* people instead of one – both of them made from the same genetic blueprint.

By contrast, fraternal twins do not have the same DNA. They come from two different eggs that have each been fertilised by different sperm cells. As a result, fraternal twins are no more closely related than normal siblings, sharing fifty per cent of their DNA.

This key difference between identical and fraternal twins can be used to examine how important genes are when it comes to various traits.

Both sets of twins grow up in similar environments, but they are not equally related, because identical twins share twice as much DNA as fraternal twins. If the identical twins are more similar than the fraternal twins when it comes to a particular trait, that is a sign that genes are important for that trait.

An interesting example of a twin study is the Minnesota Twin Study, which followed identical and fraternal twins who were adopted by different families and therefore grew up apart. The researchers expected the identical twins to differ a lot when raised apart, but were surprised by just how similarly they turned out. If you met these people, you'd probably have guessed they grew up together even though they had never met.

Nancy Segal, one of the researchers behind the study, has used the identical twins James Lewis and Jim Springer as an example. The two first met when they were in their forties, but until then they had lived strangely similar lives: they regularly went on vacation to the same beach in Florida; they both bit their nails, drove light blue Chevrolets, suffered from similar types of headaches; and had both worked part-time at a sheriff's office and at McDonald's. One twin named his son James Alan, while the other named his son James Allan. The similarities actually extended to the absurd. Both twins first married women named Linda, then divorced the Lindas and later married women named Betty. Finally, one twin divorced his Betty, so maybe the other Betty should be worried.

Now, of course, the name of your wife isn't coded in your genes. But the two brothers are evidence of just how much our genetics can influence our traits. So how about our lifespans?

One of the most prominent studies of twins and longevity was made on Danish twins born between 1870 and 1900. Here, researchers found a so-called 'heritability' for longevity of 0.26 for men and 0.23 for women. Similar results have been found in other studies: 0.25 among Amish people, 0.15 in the state of Utah and 0.33 in Sweden. The exact number isn't that important. The important thing is that the heritability is low: closer to 0 than 1.

Heritability is a somewhat technical concept, but you can understand it like this: if the heritability of a trait is 1, that means that *all* the differences between individuals are due to their genes. For instance, if the heritability of height was 1 and one person is taller than another, it means that the height difference is solely due to genetic differences between the two. If the heritability of height was 0, the difference would be solely due to the environment. So when the heritability for lifespan is 0.15–0.33, it shows that a large part of the variation in lifespan is due to something *other* than our genes.

Researchers are still doing twin studies, but they have also begun employing new study designs to untangle genes and environment. For instance, Google-owned Calico (California Life Company), has conducted a study in collaboration with Ancestry.com, which hosts more than 100 million family trees. These family trees include enormous amounts of data on the lifespans of different families, which can, of course, be analysed.

The result of the study confirmed the low heritability of longevity. That is, while your genes are highly influential on many traits, they don't matter much to how long you live.

Actually, the Calico researchers discovered that genes might be even less important than suggested by twin studies. They found that married couples – who generally are not related – have more similar lifespans than opposite-sex siblings. And, overall, there is a correlation between the lifespans of a given family and those who marry into it. This might be of some comfort if your mother-in-law has moved in and refuses to give up the ghost.

The similar lifespans of spouses probably stem from the fact that we tend to marry people who are somewhat similar to ourselves. Obviously, we don't know the life expectancy of our future partners in advance, but they are likely to be people with whom we share interests in things like diet and exercise (or lack thereof), and who have similar levels of wealth, and similar physical traits.

The point of this detail in the story is that the correlation between spouses makes it look like longevity is more genetically determined than it actually is. When researchers adjust for the effect that we marry people similar to ourselves, the heritability for longevity drops below 0.1. In other words, your lifespan is not very genetically determined at all. That's good news if you want to do something about how long you're going to live.

Heritability in history

All the studies on the heritability of lifespan are done on deceased people who were obviously born in a very different time to you and me. This might influence the results.

Height is a good analogy. In the past, your adult height was much more conditional on your environment – social class – than it is now. If you were born wealthy, you got plenty to eat, including lots of protein. If you were born poor, you'd most likely subsist on a monotonous diet and might even experience periods of hunger, all while living in crowded conditions conducive to the spread of disease. These differences meant wealthy people used to be taller than poor people, due not to their genes but to their upbringing. Today that is no longer the case. In most developed countries, even poor people get enough to eat, along with sufficient protein and childhood vaccinations. That means everyone gets the chance to grow as tall as their genetics allow. Thus, today, your adult height is much more genetically determined than it would have been in the past. Maybe the same thing will happen with longevity: the more that everyone has access to optimal conditions for a long life, the more important genetics might become.

People tend to think that if something is genetic, it is set in stone. But you should know that genes are neither magic nor fate. They're just the recipes for proteins. A genetic difference between you and me could mean that you produce a little more or a little less of a given protein, or that your version of the protein is shaped slightly differently from mine. These differences sometimes lead to variation in our traits, but they are not due to magic, just proteins.

If we learn how genetics shape differences between people, we can find ways to mimic the effect using drugs or technology. For instance, genes have an impact on your likelihood of developing poor eyesight, but today we've invented glasses, contact lenses and laser eye surgery. Eventually, we'll develop technology to make it completely irrelevant whether you're genetically inclined to near-sightedness – perhaps by mimicking the genetic mechanisms that protect some people from developing poor eyesight.

The same is true for the genetics of lifespan. While we've learned that genes have a limited impact on how long we live, their impact is not zero either. This means we can get clues to the secrets behind a long life from the genetics of long-lived people. Upon cracking these secrets, we can then design drugs to mimic the effect for the rest of us so that everyone will be able to reap the benefits.

Imagine, for example, that we discover you have a mutation in the fictional gene GENE1. At the same time, we find that you and other people who have this mutation have an increased likelihood of living a long life. When we research the mutation, we might discover that it makes you produce slightly less GENE1 protein than normal. Then, all we need to do is find a way to mimic that in the rest of us, for instance by breaking down the GENE1 protein or by using drugs that inhibit it from being produced in the first place.

To be fair, real-life biology is a bit messier than my simple theory here. The problem is that we have around 21,000 genes.

Back in the day, it was normal to say stuff like 'the gene for height' or 'the gene for obesity'. However, today we know genetics are vastly more complicated. Most of our traits are not determined by single genes, but influenced by thousands of different genes at once. For the most part, each gene – or genetic variant – only has a small impact. That means you'll have to sum up all these small effects if you want to predict something about a person. Fortunately, this *is* something we can do, by way of studies called Genome-Wide Association Studies (or GWAS). The statistics behind these studies are pretty complex, but the concept itself is simple. In a GWAS, scientists use the genomes of thousands of people in an effort to find correlations between specific genetic variants and certain traits. For example, imagine that you identify a genetic variant that is found in all blue-eyed people but not in brown-eyed people. That could be a sign that the genetic variant has something to do with eye colour. If we already know that this gene has been linked to pigment production or eye development in previous studies, the case strengthens.

Once scientists have identified tons of these small correlations, they sum them up into what is called a polygenetic risk score using statistics. Let's take a crude example: imagine that we are a pair of under-stimulated researchers who want to investigate the genes behind restlessness. We conduct a GWAS on a lot of people, and in this case we find out that the differences in restlessness are due to a thousand different genetic variants.

Then we look at you and me. In this case, we use a simple model: if a genetic variant makes a person more restless, we say +1; and if it does the opposite, we say -1. When we add all the thousand genetic variants together, I get a risk score for restlessness of +600, while you get a score of -200. In other words, I'd better get a move on with writing this book. And then you can sit back on the couch and read it.

The scientists who carry out actual GWAS for lifespan are still far from understanding the genetics of a long life. But they *have* uncovered some interesting genetic mechanisms that we can use as clues.

First, there's a clear connection to the immune system. Many genetic variants that help people live longer play some kind of role in our defence against infections.

Second, there's a connection to metabolism and growth. For example, there are genetic variants in a gene with the comprehensible name Forkhead Box O3 (FOXO3) which are correlated to living a long life. FOXO3 has a lot of jobs but one is involvement in hormonal signalling by the growth-promoting and metabolism-influencing hormones insulin and IGF-1.

Third, there's a connection to genetic variants for age-related diseases. That is, while some of the genetic variants influencing lifespan affect the ageing process itself, others affect your risk of getting an age-related disease *once* you've grown old. The most prominent of these genetic variants is in a gene called Apolipoprotein E (APOE). APOE helps transport fats, vitamins and cholesterol from the lymphatic system back into the bloodstream. But nature is fond of recycling, so it also plays a role in the nervous system and regulation of the immune system. For reasons that are still not entirely clear, APOE is a major modulator of the risk of getting Alzheimer's disease. There are three variants of the APOE gene among humans: ε2, ε3 and ε4. Most people have two versions of the 'normal' ε3 variant (one from each parent). But twenty to thirty per cent of people have one normal ε3 variant and one ε4 variant.

This increases the risk of developing Alzheimer's disease. An unlucky two per cent have *two* ε4 variants, and these people have many times the normal risk of Alzheimer's disease.

★ ★ ★

Generally, GWAS are most suitable for identifying the effects of genetic variants that are found in a large number of people. If a genetic variant is too rare, its effect can fly under the radar. That doesn't mean that rare genetic variants are unimportant for health and longevity – in fact, there's reason to believe the opposite. Fortunately, rare genetic variants with exciting effects are occasionally discovered in other circumstances.

To learn about one such case, we'll have to take a detour to the small town of Berne, Indiana. At first glance, Berne looks like most other cities in the American Midwest – a gridded street layout, big houses with nice lawns and surrounded by fields as far as the eye can see. But meet the inhabitants, and you'll notice something is different from your average Mid-westerner. Many inhabitants of Berne are dressed in modest, old-fashioned clothes and travel in horse-drawn carriages. If you get close enough to listen in on their conversations, you won't hear English but a dialect of German.

These people are Amish: a tight-knit group who practise a particular form of Christianity. Their way of life is based around hard work, modesty and eschewing most modern technology. Originally, the Amish came to North America from Germany and Switzerland in the eighteenth and nineteenth century. This is evident in that they still call every non-Amish person 'the English'. But the Amish of Europe are long gone, and now they are only found in the New World.

A hundred years ago, there were only about 5,000 Amish in the entire United States. But by the turn of the millennium, there were 166,000 and now there are more than 330,000. That's not because it's suddenly become fashionable to be Amish. In fact, it's very uncommon for outsiders to join. Instead, the Amish increase their numbers by having lots of children. As a result, the Amish of Berne mostly descend from a small group of families who moved to Indiana from Ohio in the nineteenth century. Without knowing it, one of these migrants carried a unique genetic mutation. If the person had married into the broader American population, their descendants would have spread widely, and we would probably never have discovered it. But because the person was Amish, many of their descendants are right here in Berne. In fact, some Bernese have inherited the mutation from *both* their parents because they are descended from the original carrier on both sides of their family tree.

The mutation in question is located in a gene that normally makes the protein PAI-1. It's a so-called *loss-of-function* mutation: a mutation that causes a gene to stop working. Someone who has inherited a single mutated version of the gene will produce roughly fifty per cent less PAI-1 than normal. And someone who has inherited the mutant variant from *both* parents will not make PAI-1 at all.

The reason we know about this genetic variant today is because of research from Northwestern University in Evanston, Illinois. Here, researchers have shown that increased levels of PAI-1 accelerates the ageing process in mice. Meanwhile, lowering PAI-1 is protective. Can you see where this is going?

The Amish people of Berne who carry the special PAI-1 mutation have genetically low levels of PAI-1: a genetic gift from one of their ancestors. If lower PAI-1 levels slow down ageing in mice, could it do the same in people?

The researchers set out to investigate by comparing the mutation carriers with those Amish carrying normal versions of PAI-1. Because the Amish community is tight-knit, the researchers could use family trees to go back in time and figure out who must have been carrying the mutation.

They found that the people carrying the PAI-1 mutation had indeed lived longer lives than 'normal' Amish people. That's an exciting hint that PAI-1 could affect people and mice similarly.

As we've previously discussed, the next step is to transfer this genetic gift to the rest of us. Of course, more studies are needed to confirm the effect and understand it better. But biotechnology companies are actually already working to create drugs that inhibit PAI-1. While we wait for that, we might wonder a little bit about why PAI-1 is accelerating the ageing process.

One suggestion is that PAI-1 plays an important role in something called cellular senescence. This is a special condition that some cells enter as we age, in which they hover between life and death. Call them zombie cells. The zombie cells lose their ability to divide, as well as most of their normal functions. However, for some reason they stick around and start spewing out a cocktail of molecules. These molecules – one of which is PAI-1 – can damage tissue and seem to accelerate the ageing process. So we can add 'zombie cells' to our list of biological phenomena genetically predicted to play a role in ageing.

Chapter 4

The Disadvantages of Immortality

What is half of 100? If we're talking about ageing, it's not fifty. It's ninety-three. You see, it's actually just as hard to make it from the age of ninety-three to 100 as it is to make it all the way from birth to the age of ninety-three.

This is because human ageing is exponential. If we survive birth, we enter the statistically safest part of (modern) life: being a child. At this point, we're completely immune to all of the age-related diseases that plague us later in life. Good things rarely last forever, though, and eventually we reach puberty. Then ageing starts. After we finish puberty, the risk of dying begins to increase with each additional year we live, doubling approximately every eight years. Given that the risk of death starts low, this is hardly something we notice initially. During the first decade or decade and a half after puberty, each new year doesn't feel much different to the former. But over time, the physical decline of the body becomes apparent. Eventually, the risk of death reaches many times what it was in youth. If you're lucky enough to survive the exponential onslaught of ageing and live to 100, you have the same risk of dying every single day you're alive as you had during a whole year as a twenty-five-year-old.

The reason our risk of dying increases with age like this is that our physiology slowly declines. In essence, physical decline over time is what ageing is. We all know the obvious signs, such as wrinkles and grey hair, but there is much more to ageing than what is visible on the surface. I've collected some of the changes that happen during ageing here:

	Decline
Senses, nervous system	Slower thinking; worsening memory; worsening balance; poorer vision due to less elastic eye lenses; worse eyesight in darkness; decline in sense of smell and taste.
Heart and blood vessels	Less elastic blood vessels, which raises blood pressure; weakened heart pumping function; abnormal heart rhythm becomes more common.
Muscles and bones	Less muscle mass and strength; lower endurance; lower bone density, increasing the risk of fractures; shorter height due to cartilage and vertebrae shrinking.
Outer characteristics	Skin gets thinner and drier; bruising occurs more easily; appearance of age spots, wrinkles and grey hair.
Immune system	Poorer recognition of and mobilisation against new pathogens; increased low-level activation against our own body or against nothing in particular.
Hormones	Reduction in the production of many hormones: women produce less oestrogen and progesterone and enter menopause, men produce less testosterone.

	Decline
Inner organs	Lungs: less elasticity; diminished air intake. Liver: declining ability to neutralise harmful substances like alcohol. Intestine: harmful changes in the composition of the microbiome; less integrity. Bladder: less elasticity, leading to more frequent urination.

As you might suspect from this table, the general rule is that any bodily function gets worse with age. Each form of decline doesn't happen to everyone at the same time or at the same rate. A few people never get grey hair, for instance. But pick basically any part of your physiology, and it's a safe bet it will be in a worse state in twenty years than it is now.

While some people are terribly unhappy about getting wrinkles, the real problem here is not what we look like but that all this decline drastically increases our risk of various diseases. A few people are listed as having died from 'old age', but the vast majority of people die from some sort of age-related disease. That is, a disease that only or primarily hits the elderly. This is very visible on the list of the biggest killers – here they are for the United States:

Rank	Cause of death	Percentage
1	Heart diseases	23%
2	Cancers	21%
3	Accidents	6%
4	Chronic lower respiratory diseases	6%
5	Cerebrovascular disease (especially stroke)	5%
6	Alzheimer's disease (dementia)	4%

Besides accidents, all these causes of death have one thing in common: they are overwhelmingly caused by ageing. Young people just don't get heart attacks or dementia.

We spend most of our research money on trying to better understand these diseases and on developing potential cures. But even if we were successful, that actually wouldn't be enough. For instance, imagine you found the cure to all cancers tomorrow. How much do you think your efforts would impact life expectancy? Would eradicating cancer add ten years? More?

In fact, life expectancy would only increase 3.3 years if all cancers disappeared tomorrow. If we eradicated cardiovascular diseases instead, life expectancy would go up by four years, and if we cured Alzheimer's disease, it would increase by two years. This might sound shockingly small, but the explanation is that people would simply die of something else. Their cause of death might be a disease, but the ultimate cause is ageing. A young body can keep these diseases at bay just fine because it is adept at upkeep and repair. But as we decline physically, the door is opened to age-related diseases. At first it might just be slightly ajar, but over time, it continues to open ever wider, until eventually there might even be a sign reading: 'Welcome'.

The negative side of this realisation is that age-related diseases are very hard to avoid in an old body. But the positive side is that we have a chance of shielding ourselves against many diseases at once. If the root cause of all our biggest ailments is the same, that means we can improve our resilience to all of them at once. The key is to slow down ageing. A relatively young body will be better at keeping us healthy by itself, and will be a double positive: not only do we get to spend more years in a healthy and vigorous state, we will also keep the door closed to age-related diseases for longer.

Ageing syndromes

There are certain genetic diseases that make people age much more rapidly than normal. One of these is called progeria and is characterised by a small, fragile body, hairlessness and a distinctive facial appearance. In essence, people with progeria start ageing before they've even grown up. They usually end up dying from age-related diseases such as heart attacks and strokes. But the difference is that these diseases appear dreadfully early in life: the average lifespan for people with progeria is only thirteen years.

The cause of this nasty genetic disease is a mutation in a gene making the protein lamin A. Lamin A is a part of something called the cell nucleus and when the protein is mutated, this structure ends up shaped differently than normal. For some reason, this worsens the ability to repair damage to DNA which is important to cellular health. This mechanism is shared by other genetic diseases of accelerated ageing.

While we have a good idea about the many parts of our bodies that decline during ageing, it's less clear *why* this happens in the first place. As always in biology, we should turn to Charles Darwin's theory of evolution for answers. As the biologist Theodosius Dobzhansky once said, 'Nothing in biology makes sense except in the light of evolution.' For instance, if you want to understand why a tiger has stripes, the theory of evolution has the answer: the stripes help camouflage the tiger. The tigers that are best camouflaged will catch the most prey and that means they can rear more cubs, who inherit the good camouflage from their parents. And so it continues generation after generation.

The problem is that ageing is a difficult phenomenon to make sense of when looking through the evolutionary lens, at least at first glance. How would it ever be beneficial to grow old and die? Why would animals not just evolve longer and longer lifespans so that they could continue to have offspring forever? Sure, to be successful, they would have to feed and take care of their offspring too. But there's certainly nothing to be gained by getting old. That's the surest way of getting *no* offspring. Yet, we live in a world where ageing is quite normal.

British biologist Peter Medawar has given us the most fundamental insight into why this is. He reasoned that even if most animals *could* live forever, they wouldn't. For instance, imagine that we could take our tiger from before and free it from ageing. Even if this tiger was biologically immortal, it could still get sick from an infection, become injured when prey fights back, die in an accident, get killed by another tiger or, unfortunately, end up as a trophy for some scumbag poacher. Life is dangerous in the wild, even at the top of the food chain.

The most widely accepted theories on the evolution of ageing build on this insight. Biological theorists wonder whether ageing has arisen because death is a certainty in the wild. That makes it more favourable to invest in the now than in some potential future that might never come. We've discussed this phenomenon a little already. Remember the opossums? Those living in safety on Sapelo Island had evolved longer lifespans than those living in the constant danger of the rainforest. And similarly, animals that can fly live longer than those stuck on the ground, probably because flying makes it easier to evade predators, improving the return from investing in the future.

We can envision the process with a thought experiment: imagine our tiger is born with a mutation that is detrimental from the get-go. Maybe the mutation makes the tiger bright blue. While that might look cool, it would also make it easier for the tiger's prey to see it coming. That means the blue tiger would catch less prey and have a harder time rearing its cubs. If the cubs inherited the mutation and were blue too, they would also be less successful. Eventually, the mutation would disappear.

However, what if the mutation was not detrimental immediately? Maybe instead of turning the tiger blue, the mutation makes the tiger go blind – but not until it's fifteen years old. Our tiger would be just fine for a long time and could rear lots of cubs. *If* it made it to fifteen, it would no longer be able to catch any prey, and would starve to death. But most tigers don't make it to that point anyway. This theory is called the 'mutation accumulation theory'. In short, it imagines we decline physically over time because evolution has a hard time getting rid of mutations that are only detrimental after the point where an animal would likely be dead anyway.

Now, imagine that the blindness mutation is not just *neutral* for the first fifteen years of life. What if it is *beneficial* at first? It could be that this mutation makes the tiger *better* at seeing early on at the cost of eventually losing its vision in old age. Now the mutation might help the tiger catch *more* prey and rear *more* cubs early in life. Even if the mutation dooms the tiger to eventually become blind and starve, you can imagine how this tiger could rear more cubs than a regular tiger anyway. This theory is called 'the theory of antagonistic pleiotropy' to make it easy for you to remember. In short, the theory posits that certain genetic variants can be beneficial in early life but detrimental later on. If early life is more important, these genetic variants might become common and their late-life detrimental effects would produce the physical decline that we call ageing.

★ ★ ★

The most popular theories consider ageing as a failure to properly repair damage. In essence, they propose that animals try to fight ageing but eventually run out of the necessary tools. Some researchers think this view is completely wrong. They argue that ageing is instead something *we do to ourselves*: a sort of continuation of the developmental programme that takes us from fertilised egg to baby to child to adult. This idea is usually called 'programmed ageing'. Naively, this would make sense, wouldn't it? If all animals lived forever, there'd end up being so many animals that all the food would be eaten and eventually everyone would starve. That's not a particularly clever strategy.

While this theory sounds plausible at first, it is controversial because it has serious logical and mathematical challenges. Evolution simply doesn't work on the group level like this. One of the main problems is a classic situation called 'the tragedy of the commons'. This is the same phenomenon we humans encounter when we have to take care of the environment, pay taxes or keep a shared kitchen clean. There will always be those who try to gain the benefits without contributing anything themselves.

The 'tragedy of the commons' is widespread in nature, and you might have encountered it before unknowingly. If you have ever watched nature documentaries, you might have wondered why prey animals rarely fight back. Thousands of wildebeest can be scattered by a few lions. Surely, the balance of power should be skewed the other way. No matter how strong and ferocious lions are, the many wildebeest should be able to take them down. Sometimes there could be several thousand against one! Yet every time lions come around – even just a single lion – the wildebeest flee in panic. As a result, one of them sometimes ends up getting eaten.

If the wildebeest spoke English, we could sit them down and explain the situation: 'If you cooperate, you have the upper hand. You can kill the lions by teaming up on them and then be free from predators.' The wildebeest would obviously be swayed by our logic and make a plan to defend themselves. Then, during the next lion attack, they would bravely fight back. Several wildebeest might get injured, but their numbers would make them victorious in the end. From then on, the wildebeest would be free of their tormentors.

Occasionally, the wildebeest would have to fight new lion packs, but by cooperating, they would be able to much improve their lives.

However, as in any group, there will be a coward among the wildebeest. This guy likes the newfound safety as much as everyone else. But he doesn't feel like putting his own life on the line – the others can do that. So, the next time lions attack, the coward makes sure to end up at the back of the defence. That way, he doesn't risk anything, while the other wildebeest keep the herd safe.

The brave wildebeest at the front are occasionally wounded and some even die. The coward, on the other hand, always manages to stay safe. He lives far longer than the average wildebeest and has more offspring as a result. Some of the offspring are also cowards and make sure to stay safe at the back like their father. As a result, the cowardly wildebeest have more offspring through the generations than the brave wildebeest. They only think of themselves and stay safe by never risking anything for others. However, this means that eventually, the whole herd consists of cowards. When this happens, the clever defence tactic fails and it's every wildebeest for itself again.

In our own society, we've invented social mechanisms that make it harder to cheat in this way. We'll punish people trying to evade taxes, go after companies that pollute the environment, or gossip about the person who tries to get out of cleaning a shared kitchen. But even with our cultural adaptations in hand, it is still difficult to take care of the environment, collect taxes or keep a shared kitchen clean. Nature isn't nearly as lucky as we humans are – it can't foresee problems or think about them rationally. Evolution is a blind walk in nature and the optimal solution to the 'tragedy of the commons' is often to be a coward yourself.

This is why programmed ageing would be challenging. Even if we imagine that it could somehow evolve (which would be very unlikely in the first place), it would be confronted with the 'tragedy of the commons'. Programming ageing into the genes of an organism means that the programme would be vulnerable to mutations. At one point, an individual would be born with a dysfunctional ageing programme. This individual would then be biologically immortal and have a massive advantage. It would have much more offspring than the other members of its species that dutifully age and die. And eventually this immortal creature would become the common ancestor for all of us.

So given that we're not all immortal right now, programmed ageing seems unlikely. The reason I'm mentioning it anyway is that there are a lot of examples from nature and the laboratory that sure *look* like something of the sort. For instance:

- Queen and worker bees have the same genes. Whether a larva becomes a queen or a worker simply depends on the food and care the larva gets. Yet despite their identical genetic blueprint, there is a huge difference between the lifespan of a queen and that of a worker bee. A worker bee lives for a few weeks while the queen can live for years. The same goes for ants.

- As we've learned, female octopuses guard their eggs full-time, then die within a few days of the hatching. However, if you remove a particular gland called the optic gland, the mother will stay alive. Removing one of the two optic glands, prolongs the life of the octopus a few weeks while removing *both* optic glands means more than forty more weeks of life.

- In the 1980s, American scientist Tom Johnson discovered that you can prolong the life of the laboratory worm *C. elegans* by shutting down a gene dubbed age-1. At first, scientists thought the worms lived longer because disabling age-1 made them shift resources from reproduction towards upkeep and repair. But later it turned out that worms with disabled age-1 get just as many offspring as normal worms. It appears there are no drawbacks – losing this gene simply extends the worm's lifespan. Since the age-1 finding, scientists have found many other genes that can be disabled in *C. elegans* and similarly extend lifespan with no apparent downsides. That is very unexpected according to the conventional theories.

Maybe all this speculation just sounds like academics arguing with each other for the sake of arguing, but actually, the question of who is right is vital to the fight against ageing. Understanding what ageing *is* determines what our approach should be when looking for ways to combat it. If ageing is the body failing to repair itself, as the conventional theories say, then the solution is damage repair. We should identify all the different ways in which our bodies decline and fix each of them, one at a time. If, on the other hand, ageing is programmed, that implies a much easier solution: rewind the programme. We already understand a lot about how the early developmental programme works: how we go from conception to a baby, and from child to adult. If ageing follows a similar kind of programme, we don't need to fix the damage that accumulates in old age. We just need to understand the ageing programme and wind it back. Then, our bodies would become biologically young again and take care of the damage by themselves, like young bodies normally do.

As it is probably clear by now, we're not in a position to choose between these two options yet. You can bet on one of them when deciding what to research or invest in. But for trying to combat ageing right now, the rational thing to do is to keep our minds open to all possibilities.

Part II

SCIENTISTS' DISCOVERIES

Chapter 5
What Doesn't Kill You . . .

Take the subway in my hometown of Copenhagen and you'll probably see some ad for a new smoothie absolutely *packed* with antioxidants. The same goes for sketchy diet supplements sold by 'influencers' and other online pyramid schemes. However, the love story between antioxidants and health supplements actually began under somewhat more serious circumstances.

In the 1950s – a few years after the first nuclear bombs were dropped in Japan – scientists were understandably concerned about the effects of radioactivity on the human body. As always, mice had to suffer so that humans won't. Scientists found that exposing mice to high, but not lethal, levels of radioactive radiation accelerated the ageing process. When irradiated, the mice would develop age-related diseases sooner than normal, and they would also die earlier.

One reason radioactivity harms mice is that it creates something called free radicals in cells. These are highly reactive molecules that will damage other molecules when bumping into them. You can imagine free radicals as a bull in a china shop. When the cells of any animal are exposed to radioactivity, the bull goes on a rampage inside the cells. Scientists call the total damage done by the bull 'oxidative stress'. So mice that are exposed to radiation have 'high oxidative stress'.

This is where *anti*oxidants come into the picture. The 'anti' refers to the ability to *neutralise* free radicals and you can think of antioxidants as a sedative to our bull. Because of this, the radiation researchers discovered that they could use antioxidants to protect their mice from the harmful effects of radioactivity. And their conclusion was that antioxidants help irradiated animals live longer.

The interesting thing is, though, that free radicals don't just arise in cells that are irradiated. They're actually produced as a normal by-product of metabolism in all of us. This means your cells are constantly at the mercy of the rampaging bull. Scientists knew this and started speculating. What if free radicals are not just the cause of *radiation-induced* ageing? What if they are the cause of *normal* ageing as well? This theory is called the 'free radical theory of ageing'.

Simply put, the theory posits there is a sort of Faustian bargain in our metabolism: it is what keeps us alive, but it's also what ensures that we age and die because it produces free radicals.

The theory fits the fact that free radicals are obviously causing damage, that old people have higher levels of oxidative stress than young people, and that excess oxidative stress has been linked to all age-related diseases. But fortunately, the theory also comes with an easy solution: use antioxidants to tame the rampaging bull.

This idea is many decades old now, and it has been thoroughly tested in clinical trials.

In fact, it's been tested so much that researchers can do what is known as a *meta-analysis*: a huge study that analyses the data from several separate studies as one.

In one such meta-analysis – composed of sixty-eight studies and 230,000 subjects – researchers investigated whether dietary supplements with antioxidants help people live longer.

Their conclusion: people who take antioxidant supplements die *earlier*. They aren't protected against age-related diseases either. In fact, it looks like antioxidant supplements will *promote* the growth and spread of certain cancers rather than limit them.

★ ★ ★

In the fall of 1991, eight scientists were locked inside a huge futuristic greenhouse in Oracle, Arizona. Biosphere 2, as the building is called, was to be their home for the next two years. Their mission: to provide themselves with food, water, oxygen and the rest of life's necessities without any outside help.

This grand experiment was done to test whether we can create a full ecosystem from scratch. On Earth, we're lucky to already be a part of just that: nature provides us with all of life's necessities, and if we treat her properly, she will be able to take care of us for a long time. However, when some of us eventually leave Earth to settle other planets, we'll need to establish new ecosystems from scratch to provide for us.

As you might know, one of the most important parts of Earth's ecosystems is trees. Not only do trees provide oxygen, they're also living quarters for countless species and can be used as building material if needed. For these reasons, scientists envisioned trees as a pillar of their new ecosystem and planted plenty of trees in Biosphere 2. Trees live a long time, as we've learned, so a few years should be no problem, right?

The trees in Biosphere 2 did get off to a good start. Because of the favourable conditions inside the giant greenhouse, they grew rapidly. But before the grand experiment was over, many of the trees were already dead. What were they missing?

Not care and nurture. Quite the contrary, actually. What the trees of Biosphere 2 were missing was *stress*. More specifically, they were missing the stress that the wind normally subjects them to.

You see, although the wind is one of the worst enemies of a tree, it turns out trees can't do without it. The tireless onslaught of the wind makes trees build resilience and grow strong. Remove the wind, and trees become so weak that they eventually topple under their own weight.

Think back to the story of free radicals and antioxidants. Why do people die earlier when they take antioxidant supplements? For the same reason trees die without the wind. *The stressor keeps the organism strong.*

This biological phenomenon – getting stronger from adversity – is called *hormesis*. The most relatable example in humans is exercise. You might think that the actual act of, say, going for a run is what is healthy. But think about what actually happens while you're running. Your heart rate and blood pressure skyrocket. With every step, your muscles and bones are burdened and strained. And because exercise requires energy, your metabolism shoots up, *which increases the production of free radicals.* That's right, exercise directly leads to the production of harmful molecules. However, in the long term, exercise makes you healthier. That's because the beating serves as a message. *You need to get stronger.*

Ironically, some of the 'messengers' that start this process are free radicals. That means antioxidants *interfere* with the process of getting stronger and healthier from exercise. Fitness influencer sales pitches notwithstanding, antioxidants can cancel out some of the benefits you get from your workouts.

While exercise is the best-known example of hormesis, there are many more in the biological world. In fact, hormesis is a fundamental part of the story of life on Earth. You can safely count on the fact that your ancestors took hit after hit after hit, including miserable periods of hunger, back-breaking work, poisoning, fist fights and life-or-death escapes from predators. Life has always been challenging and for that reason challenges have become a necessity for us.

One of the best examples of the ubiquity of hormesis in nature comes from research into the toxic chemical element arsenic. Arsenic has been called the 'king of poisons' and 'poison of kings' because it is easy to acquire, odour- and tasteless, and can be used to kill a person. As a result, it has always been a favourite among ambitious royals and various psychopaths around the world.

In recent times, arsenic has, unfortunately, also become a contaminant of drinking water in several parts of the world, so researchers have undertaken studies to investigate how the toxin affects laboratory animals.

When researchers give high amounts of arsenic to the worm *C. elegans,* the poison lives up to its reputation and is a sure-fire killer. However, if the worms are instead exposed to a fixed low dose, they actually live *longer* than usual. At the same time, they also become more resistant to heat stress and other poisonous substances. Why? Hormesis, of course. While arsenic is poisonous, low doses function as a survivable stressor that makes the worms raise their defensive capabilities.

Other researchers have even succeeded in prolonging the life of *C. elegans* using a *pro-oxidant.* The opposite of an antioxidant, this is something that *increases* oxidative stress. It would be like doping our metaphorical bull in a china shop with caffeine pills and giving it a smack on the backside. In their experiment, the researchers found that they could reliably increase the lifespan of *C. elegans* using the pro-oxidant herbicide paraquat. However, if they also gave the worms antioxidants, then the damage was neutralised and the worms lived no longer than usual.

I know it sounds insane that the 'king of poisons' or a powerful herbicide can be beneficial to an organism in any way. But welcome to the world of biology.

We obviously don't have clinical trials where humans intentionally take arsenic, herbicides or other harmful substances. But there are in fact real-world parallels that showcase hormesis in humans, too.

One example is an accident that occurred in Taiwan in the 1980s. Back then, Taiwan was in the middle of an economic boom of epic proportions. As one of the Four Asian Tigers, its capital city of Taipei saw construction like never before. And in the fervour, some steel was contaminated with the radioactive cobalt-60. This steel was later used to build over 1,700 apartments, but no one noticed until the 1990s – and by then, it was too late.

It's estimated that about 10,000 people lived in the radioactive apartments before they were torn down. These people were exposed to daily radioactivity far above normal levels, and this was a cause for concern because radiation is known to damage DNA, which can lead to cancer. However, doctors were perplexed when examining the residents' medical histories. It turns out the apartment residents had *fewer* cases of virtually all types of cancer than comparable Taiwanese people.

This phenomenon has been noted elsewhere, too. Among American shipyard workers, those who work with nuclear submarines have a lower mortality rate than workers at normal shipyards. In the general US population, those living in areas with higher-than-usual background radiation live longer than average. And among physicians, radiologists – who are exposed to ionising radiation – live longer than other doctors and have a lower risk of cancer.

Let me just make absolutely clear that I do *not* recommend exposing yourself to radiation or ingesting various toxins. That would be a waste of good genes. We have no idea what levels could potentially be hormetic but we do know what happens if you exceed these levels: pain and a horrible death. You see, hormesis is all about the dose. It's healthier to challenge your body by jogging than never exercising at all. But you can also exercise *too much* – this is called overtraining. Similarly, trees grow stronger when exposed to the wind. But if the wind becomes *too strong*, it will instead knock the tree over or break it in half. We only benefit from a stressor if the resulting damage doesn't exceed our ability to repair ourselves.

It is also important to remember that not everything that is harmful or a stressor is necessarily hormetic. You will not get smarter by banging your head against the wall or improve your lung function by smoking, for instance. The stressors we react to positively are primarily those we have evolved to resist.

★ ★ ★

Outside of exercise, one of the best places to find hormesis is in our food. That's not because pizzas or doughnuts are secretly healthy if you just find the right dose. No, the place to look for hormetic substances is actually in the plants we eat.

You see, like so many other living things, plants prefer to live rather than get eaten. It's just a little harder when you can't run away from those trying to eat you. So that leaves plants with a single option for survival – fight. Some plants do this by having intimidating thorns, iron-hard shells or stinging needles. But what most plants have in common is that they also wage chemical warfare against their enemies. And we're on that list.

It might be easy to eat a plant-based diet today, but as a Stone Age person you really had to know what you were doing. An incredible number of plants are poisonous in one way or another. Wild almonds, for instance, contain cyanide, one of the most toxic chemicals we know of. And raw cashews contain the same toxic substance as poison ivy (which is neutralised by the time they reach the supermarket, so don't worry).

Even the plants that aren't toxic to us (and that we regularly eat) are often toxic to other animals. Just think of chocolate and other cocoa products, which are toxic to both cats and dogs. And most of the plants we *do* eat still have some fight in them. Take pineapple – have you ever had a little pain in your mouth or tongue after eating one? If you have, there's a good reason for it: pineapples contain protein-degrading enzymes. These can be used to tenderise meat, but it's not so pleasant when you *are* the meat. As soon as you eat the pineapple, its enzymes will essentially start digesting you by breaking down proteins in your mouth. We're too big for this to be a deterrent, but it's a hefty weapon against smaller animals.

Another good example is chilli. Chillies contain a compound called capsaicin, which is what makes your mouth burn when you eat them. When a mammal eats the chilli pepper, the seeds are crushed and capsaicin is released. This ensures the mammal won't eat chillies again anytime soon. Birds, on the other hand, swallow the seeds whole, feel fine and can spread the plant far and wide. It's a clever evolutionary system.

The fact that plants are not just passively willing to get eaten has often been overlooked when discussing their health benefits. We have overwhelming evidence that including lots of plants in your diet is healthy. But scientists are still discussing why this is. There are, of course, numerous reasons but hormesis is certainly one. For instance, compounds called polyphenols have long been hailed as one of the prime reasons plants are healthy. It was once thought that it had to be because polyphenols help us in some way – perhaps by being antioxidants? But the truth is that many polyphenols are a little bit toxic to us and work by hormesis. Studies show that our bodies react to polyphenols by trying to neutralise and get rid of them, for instance, by upregulating a gene called Nrf2, which controls a wide range of cellular defence mechanisms. This gene is also upregulated after radioactive radiation.

Hormesis in animals

Long-lived birds don't have less oxidative stress than short-lived birds. And naked mole-rats have at least as much oxidative stress as their shorter-lived cousins, mice. In general, naked mole-rats seem to live a long time not because they are stress-free but because they are sublimely equipped to deal with stressors. Whether it's exposure to DNA-harming chemicals, low oxygen levels, ingestion of heavy metals, or exposure to extreme heat, naked mole-rats fare far better than mice. It seems the secret to a long life is not to live without difficult times, but to be able to withstand the onslaught.

You can consider eating lots of plants as a safe and superior alternative to ingesting toxins. How about a safe and superior alternative to moving into a radioactive apartment? One idea would be to get high up in the mountains. The atmosphere is thinner at high altitudes, and that means you're less protected from the sun's UV rays as well as being exposed to cosmic radiation. I can attest to that as a pale inhabitant of one of the flattest countries in the world having got the sunburn of a lifetime at an altitude of five kilometres.

It might not be surprising to you anymore, but despite the radiation and harsh conditions – or because of them – people who live at high altitudes tend to live longer and experience fewer age-related diseases than those who live at sea level. This has been noted in both Austria, Switzerland, Greece and California.

At higher altitudes, there are also lower oxygen levels than at sea level, and this too might play a role as a health-promoting stressor. At least, one of the reactions your cells have to both radiation exposure and low oxygen levels is the production of something called heat shock proteins. As the name suggests, these proteins were originally discovered in connection to high heat, but it turns out they are part of a more general suit of cellular protective mechanisms. Just as we have seen before, this illustrates that hormesis is often far-reaching. The response to one stressor will tend to improve resilience against other stressors, too.

You can think of heat shock proteins as a sort of protein superhero that helps other proteins. When cells are damaged by some kind of stressor, many proteins end up in the wrong shape. But heat shock proteins help them recover their form and function so that they don't turn into cellular junk.

Interestingly, the namesake of the heat shock proteins, heat shock, is not restricted to laboratory animals. It's an integrated part of Nordic culture in the form of the sauna. The homeland of the sauna, Finland, has blessed us with more sauna studies than we could ever have asked for. And in these studies, sauna use tends to correlate with various health benefits – a lower risk of cardiovascular diseases and a longer lifespan, for instance. Heat shock proteins probably play a role in these health benefits, but there are also other beneficial effects from sauna use, such as lowered blood pressure. (When it comes to the sauna, there is a small 'but' to bear in mind, though: men who want to be able to have children should not spend too much time in the sauna, for the same reason that it can be a bad idea to spend long stints in hot tubs, or to sit with a laptop in your lap.)

Besides heat exposure, another integral part of Nordic culture is cold exposure in the form of winter swimming. Actually, the two are often undertaken in a single session, with a cold dip interchanged with sauna stints. We don't have the same amount of data on the benefits of cold exposure as we do on sauna use. But it is easy to imagine cold exposure could also have long-term health benefits. For one, it activates something called 'brown fat', which works in the opposite way to normal fat. It's for *burning* energy, not storing it – in doing so it warms us up. And interestingly, it turns out that many long-lived species have naturally increased activity in their brown fat tissue. Proof or not, the hardcore winter swimmers I know swear by the effect. They notice an increase in energy, fewer sick days and report a general feeling of wellbeing. After the swim, that is.

Chapter 6

Does Size Matter?

The year 1492 was among the most eventful ones in the area that has today become Spain. Two days into the new year, the Muslim Emir of Granada surrendered to the Catholic King Ferdinand of Aragon and Queen Isabella of Castile. The surrender ended the centuries-long *reconquista*, in which the Catholic kingdoms of the north slowly regained their homeland from Muslim conquerors.

Two weeks after the decisive battle, the two monarchs met with a merchant from Genoa in present-day Italy. For years, this merchant, Christopher Columbus, had been requesting they support his idea: finding a sea route to Asia by sailing *west*. In return for their support and funding, he promised that the new route would bring the monarchs and their kingdoms enormous wealth.

We don't know why – maybe it was the optimism of victory – but that year, the monarchs agreed to fund Columbus's journey. Soon, three Spanish ships set sail and headed west across the Atlantic. After a long journey, they landed on the American continent as the first Europeans since the Vikings.

Meanwhile, King Ferdinand and Queen Isabella were also plenty occupied at home. After centuries of religious and territorial conflict on their peninsula, they wanted their new kingdoms to be completely Christian. In what's called the Alhambra Decree, the Spanish Jews were given an ultimatum: convert to Christianity or leave the country. Some chose their home over their faith and became converts or *conversos*. The rest made the opposite choice and ventured out in search of a new home.

The following year, Columbus and his crew returned from the Americas. They initially thought they had been to Asia, but over time, it became clear that the Spanish had reached a continent that was unknown to Europeans at the time. Soon, the Spanish colonisation of the Americas was underway. Spaniards from all walks of life – farmers, criminals, families, priests, soldiers, nobles and prostitutes – set off towards the new continent. Among those emigrants were also *conversos*, descendants of the converted Jews. Despite their conversion to Christianity, they were still discriminated against in Spain, and hoped to become free in the New World.

★ ★ ★

In 1958, the Israeli physician Zvi Laron and his colleagues began studying a special group of patients. All of them had dwarfism, though not in the way you might imagine it. Sure, Laron's patients were short, about 120cm (4 feet) tall. But they didn't have the body proportions associated with the most common form of dwarfism, such as short limbs and a proportionally larger torso and head. The patients simply looked like scaled-down versions of regular people.

Laron and his colleagues spent eight years carefully investigating the cause of this new syndrome before they could share their results. It turns out patients with Laron syndrome, as it is now called, are short because of a genetic mutation involving growth hormone. The defect is not found in the hormone itself, though. In fact, patients with Laron syndrome have quite a lot of growth hormone in their blood. The reason they don't grow taller is a defect in the growth hormone *receptor*. That is, the receptor that is responsible for the cell sensing and responding to the growth hormone. You can appreciate the mechanism through an analogy. Imagine the cell as a castle ruled by a powerful, but paranoid, nobleman. The nobleman won't let outsiders in, so if someone wants to reach him, they will have to shout their message to the guards in the castle tower. Under normal circumstances, the guards will go to the nobleman and recite the message so that he can give his orders. But if the guards are deaf, they won't hear the message, no matter how loudly outsiders try to scream at them. And then the nobleman will never receive it or respond.

In a similar way, the signal from growth hormone never reaches the cells of patients with Laron syndrome. Their defective growth hormone receptors mean growth hormone can float around in the blood at high concentrations without ever inducing growth.

★ ★ ★

Nearly 500 years after the Spanish first set foot in the Americas, a newly trained physician in Ecuador was pondering a mystery from his childhood. Jaime Guevara-Aguirre, as he is called, remembered meeting a curious number of people with dwarfism while growing up. With his newly acquired medical degree in hand, he was ready to find out why. The quest took Guevara-Aguirre back to his home region in the mountainous Loja province. Here, he had to travel on horseback to reach his desired destination: some remote villages deep in the mountains. The trouble proved worthwhile, though, and just as he'd recalled, Guevara-Aguirre encountered several people who looked like miniature versions of their relatives.

The explanation is that all these people had Laron syndrome. Without knowing it, they were distant relatives of Zvi Laron's patients in Israel. You see, the Ecuadoreans with Laron syndrome are partly descended from the Spanish Jews who converted to Christianity and later took part in the colonisation of the Americas. Zvi Laron's patients in Israel, on the other hand, are descended from the Spanish Jews who made the opposite choice, leaving Spain to keep their religion. While the winding paths of history have driven the two groups apart, the Laron discovery has pulled them right back together. We now know that one of their ancestors must have had a mutation in the growth hormone receptor. To actually get Laron syndrome, though, it is not enough to inherit a single defective version of the growth hormone receptor. If this happens, there's still a functional version from the other parent and the affected person will just be a few centimetres shorter than normal. But inherit defective growth hormone receptors from *both* your parents and you have no functional ones. *Then* you get Laron syndrome. This is the reason the syndrome is rare in Israel today. It's unlikely for two people to both carry the mutation and pass it on to the same child. In the remote villages of the Loja province, though, Laron syndrome is much more common. The reason is the same one we saw among the Amish of Berne. The region is isolated and was originally settled by a small group of people. Later, the population grew from these few people intermarrying again and again while expanding their numbers.

So Jaime Guevara-Aguirre had found the perfect place to study Laron syndrome. He wasted no time, and before long he made a remarkable discovery. It turns out people with Laron syndrome almost never get cancer. In the entire time these people have been studied, only a single cancer case has been noted. Cancer is characterised by excessive growth (of the tumour), so it sounds reasonable that lack of growth signals would be protective. But people with Laron syndrome actually don't get other age-related diseases either. They're protected against cardiovascular diseases, dementia and diabetes. Heck, they don't even get acne. And all this is despite many Laron people in Ecuador being overweight and subsisting on diets high in processed foods. It's as if the Laron mutation protects them from disease, even in the face of poor habits.

★ ★ ★

In an effort to study Laron syndrome, researchers have bred mice whose growth hormone receptors are also impaired. Just like their human equivalents, these mice are much smaller than average, but have regular proportions. And, like the humans with Laron syndrome, the Laron mice are also remarkably healthy. In fact, they live much longer than regular mice. Various studies have found that their lifespans are between sixteen and fifty-five per cent longer than normal. If you remember our rule about size and lifespan, this should be no surprise. Large animal species generally live longer than small ones – but within each species, the smallest individuals tend to live the longest. And the Laron mice are about as small a mouse as you can get. Another contender would be Ames dwarf mice that I briefly mentioned earlier. As the name suggests, these mice are tiny too, and they actually have the species lifespan record for mice. Ames dwarf mice are small for a similar reason to Laron mice, though. They have a defect in the pituitary gland just below the brain that means they don't produce growth hormone at all.

So, how about humans? If smaller individuals tend to live longer in the animal kingdom, does that mean tall people should be worried? Well, the French woman Jeanne Calment holds the world record for longest lifespan at 122 years and 164 days. That is one unusual trait of Calment's; another is that she was only 150cm (4 feet 11 inches) tall. Just below her on the longevity record list is American Sarah Knauss, who was 140cm (4 feet 7 inches) tall, while further down are Marie-Louise Meilleur, who was the same height as Calment, and Emma Morano, who was 152cm (4 feet 10 inches) tall. To be fair, all of these women were born at a time when people were generally shorter than we are today. But when learning about the longest-lived people, you'll quickly notice that they would make an extremely poor basketball team – even in their own time.

If we zoom out to population level, the association between height and longevity remains. For instance, remember how we learned that Northern Europeans tend to die earlier than Southern Europeans and East Asians, even though Northern European countries are richer? Well, Northern Europeans are also taller than Southern Europeans and East Asians, so maybe that explains it.

Another example is that American sociologists used to ponder what is called the Hispanic Paradox. That is, Hispanic Americans tend to live longer than white Americans, even though white Americans 'should' live longer on paper: they're richer, more highly educated and have slightly lower obesity rates. But Hispanic Americans are shorter.

A third example is the Blue Zones. There's Okinawa, which is among the shortest prefectures in Japan, a country whose inhabitants are already among the shortest in the developed world. And there's Sardinia, which is one of the shortest regions in Europe. The average height for men in Sardinia is 168cm (5 feet 6 inches), several inches shorter than the Italian average, and almost half a foot shorter than the tallest populations in Europe. We know the Sardinian stature is genetic in origin, and interestingly, one of the culprits is the Laron mutation, which is carried by 0.87 per cent of Sardinians. This is among the highest frequencies of the mutation in the world, though obviously lower than among the Ecuadoreans of the Loja province.

Now, all of this doesn't mean that you're destined to die early if you're tall. Or alternatively, that you can expect your shortness to carry you. These things are *averages*. There are lots of short people who die early and lots of tall people who live long and healthy lives. But *on average*, there is definitely something about the connection between size and lifespan. And that means it can teach us something about ageing.

★ ★ ★

It's obviously not height itself that ages people. If we compressed you really hard to make you shorter, you wouldn't suddenly live longer – probably the opposite. So what is it that makes short people live longer than tall people? For one, large people have more cells than small people. That means they have more cells that can become cancerous and thus have a slightly increased cancer risk. However, that is nowhere near enough to account for this phenomenon. Instead, the explanation is probably that height is a sign of how you respond to growth signals. Tallness could mean you have stronger growth signals than others or that you are more responsive to them.

So to discover the secrets of a long life, we need to head down the rabbit hole that is growth signalling. As we saw in the Ames dwarf mice, we start just below the brain in the pituitary gland. This gland releases growth hormone, but despite the name, growth hormone is not actually responsible for growth – not directly, at least. Instead, growth hormone travels to the liver, where it binds to growth hormone receptors. This binding makes the liver produce *another* hormone called IGF-1 (insulin-like growth factor 1), and it is IGF-1 that actually makes stuff grow. This means Laron syndrome can be treated by synthetic IGF-1, not by growth hormone.

So IGF-1 brings us one step further down the rabbit hole. We can verify that we're going in the right direction by looking at laboratory organisms. The various long-lived dwarf mice we discussed previously all have low IGF-1 levels. Meanwhile, one of the best ways to prolong life in the worm *C. elegans* is to inhibit the worm's own version of IGF-1. And then, of course, we have human evidence from the Laron patients. Unfortunately, these people have a high rate of deaths in accidents because of their small size, so we don't actually know if they live longer than others. However, as they're protected against age-related diseases, it would be no surprise.

Now, obviously it's not certain that you would trade in some of your height in return for a longer life; I guess it depends on where your priorities lie. But blocking IGF-1 could still be useful. Age-related diseases happen much later in life than growth, so it is possible we could block IGF-1 in old age and get both stature and a decreased risk of cancer and other age-related diseases. Perhaps even a longer life.

Ironically, growth hormone – and by extension, the IGF-1 it creates – has been dubbed an 'anti-ageing' cure since the 1980s. You see, growth hormone has been a popular 'supplement' among bodybuilders since its discovery because it promotes muscle growth. But some older bodybuilders discovered that the injections did much more than that. The growth hormone also made them feel young and bursting with energy – and thus the idea of using growth hormone to combat ageing was born.

Before decrying the irony, it's important to remember that feeling young and energetic is valuable on its own. But aside from this, there *are* some things the growth hormone proponents are right about. IGF-1 definitely has positive aspects, even when it comes to ageing. It promotes growth of muscles and bones, which is beneficial in old age. Sure, it's not healthy to look like the real-world equivalent of He-Man, but maintaining muscle and bone strength in old age is important. In addition, IGF-1 stimulates immune function, which is also something we want, because our immune systems tend to weaken and lose their punch as we age. This is bad news for fighting infections and cancer.

So clearly, there's something more going on here than simply 'IGF-1 = bad'. The problem is that IGF-1 is one of those general-purpose hormones with a ton of functions. Our bodies are very fond of recycling like this. For instance, the hormone oxytocin is involved in bonding between people but is also used in hospitals to induce childbirth because it makes the muscles of the uterus contract.

Because IGF-1 has so many functions we have to be able to tell them apart before we can learn which ones promote ageing. Some researchers have tried to do this in a clever study using *C. elegans*. The researchers discovered that it is only helpful to block IGF-1 in the nervous system of the worms. If they blocked it in muscle tissue, the worms would die *sooner* than normal. So all this suggests broadly blocking IGF-1 is not the best idea. Maybe in the future, researchers will succeed in making therapies that target IGF-1 at just the right time and in just the right place to be rejuvenating. But given the mixed signals here, it is a hard target for experimenting. Instead, we should continue down the rabbit hole.

Chapter 7

The Secrets of Easter Island

Imagine that you're looking out at the ocean from a remote little island. Below, the waves beat rhythmically against the rocks. If you turn around, you will be greeted by a golden, rocky landscape with sporadic outcroppings of grass. There are no trees. Instead, the landscape is dominated by huge stone sculptures that keep watch over the island as if to guard its inhabitants.

The isolation is palpable – the nearest inhabited island is nearly 2,000km (1,242 miles) distant, and the mainland is even further away. You're on Easter Island, where 8,000 inhabitants live surrounded by the Pacific Ocean as far as the eye can see. This isolated island may not be the most obvious place for our quest. There are no universities or biomedical laboratories, and the few scientists around are mostly interested in the stone sculptures called *Moai*. Myths claim that these huge people of stone have supernatural powers that can help fulfil any wish. Maybe someone once asked them for a longer life, because it turns out one of the ingredients is hiding in the very soil of Easter Island.

We know of this secret because a Canadian research expedition travelled to the isolated island in the 1960s to examine the soil. The Canadians were intrigued that islanders never got tetanus even though they were walking around barefoot. Tetanus is caused by a bacterial infection and is often associated with stepping on something sharp or a rupture of the skin. The bacterium involved releases a toxin into the bloodstream that makes all muscles contract to the point of being extremely painful, immobilising and even deadly.

Using soil samples from around Easter island, the Canadian researchers confirmed that there was no tetanus bacteria to be found. After that, their soil samples could easily have been thrown out or forgotten at the back of some dark university freezer. But instead, they ended up at the pharmaceutical company Ayerst Pharmaceutical, where their true secret was revealed: a bacterium called *Streptomyces hygroscopicus*. This bacterium produces a special molecule, which has been named 'rapamycin' after the indigenous name for Easter Island, Rapa Nui.

Rapamycin is actually a weapon used by this bacterium in the ancient battle against fungi. The molecule blocks – or inhibits – a specific protein complex in fungi called mTOR. Unfortunately, mTOR is not named after the God of Thunder, but just means 'mechanistic target of rapamycin'. Despite the boring name, though, mTOR is a big deal. It is a kind of central command in the cell controlling growth. So the bacterium has an ingenious weapon at its disposal. Rapamycin dampens the growth of its enemy, fungi, and this gives the bacterium a leg-up in the fight for resources.

You and I don't look much like fungi but they're actually a distant relative of ours. That means we share many proteins with fungi, among them the ones making up mTOR. In fact, mTOR is the next step down our rabbit hole of growth signalling. First, we had growth hormone – inhibit it and prolong life. Then we reached IGF-1 – again, inhibit it and prolong life. And now we have mTOR. When IGF-1 binds to cell receptors, one of the main consequences is that the mTOR complex is activated. That means mTOR 'wakes up' and can in turn initiate many processes in the cell related to growth. For instance, production of new proteins and uptake of nutrients. Now, our version of mTOR is not identical to the ones in fungi but rapamycin still works the same way. So maybe you can guess where I'm going here. When scientists give rapamycin to laboratory animals it inhibits the growth-promoting mTOR and in turn extends their lives. Mice on rapamycin actually live twenty per cent longer than usual. That's a pretty solid lifespan extension for a drug. If we transferred that twenty per cent difference directly to humans, that would be the difference between me dying while I was still a kindergartner, and me staying alive to write this book you're now reading.

★ ★ ★

Rapamycin is actually already approved for use in humans. The reason we're not all using this drug to fight ageing already is that it was developed for a completely different purpose. The researchers from Ayerst Pharmaceutical knew nothing about its effects on ageing, but they discovered that rapamycin can be helpful during organ transplants. At high doses, rapamycin inhibits the immune system, which helps lower the risk that immune cells will recognise the new organ as something foreign and attack it with deadly consequences.

The good news is that this means rapamycin has been used for many years and we have ample safety data. We know there are no crazy side effects like brain damage or exploding. But that said, rapamycin at the doses used for organ transplantations is harsh on the body and not likely to be beneficial. Weakening the immune system is not good if you want to live a long life. Transplant patients using high doses of rapamycin are at a greater risk of infections, and, as the immune system is fighting with one arm tied behind its back, infections tend to become more severe as well.

Lower doses of rapamycin are more promising, though. Studies show that low doses can even *improve* immune function, perhaps due to hormesis. Despite this, we don't know whether low doses of rapamycin can prolong life in humans. Yet. Several companies and research groups are currently working on various ways to find out. Most are trying to optimise rapamycin in some way, for instance by enhancing the effect, optimising dosing or working to limit side effects, all with the aim of making rapamycin the first widely used anti-ageing drug. Whether all this effort will pay off, time will tell. But besides companies and research groups, there are actually already various self-experimentalists who use rapamycin in an effort to fight ageing. Self-reports on the internet are positive but we probably wouldn't hear about it if they weren't. Unless you're a little crazy, rapamycin is really more of a Hail Mary for now – that is, the long and risky last-minute pass in American football that is only fit for times of desperation. Instead, we should continue down our rabbit hole.

Dogs should live forever

The sad thing about our best friends is that they don't live very long. If we're trying to extend our own lives, why not our dogs' lives too? In fact, dogs are a great opportunity for ageing research. It is much cheaper and easier for scientists to set up animal trials than human ones, which means we can catch two birds with one stone. We can help our best friends live longer and at the same time get valuable lessons for future studies in humans.

In one dog study, for instance, scientists are giving rapamycin to forty family dogs. So far, the results are great, and the dogs have improved heart function compared to the beginning of the trial. Whether they will also live longer, time will tell.

Chapter 8
The One to Unite Them All

In 2016, the Nobel Prize in Medicine was awarded to Japanese biologist Yoshinori Ohsumi. His contribution: research into something in our cells called 'autophagy'. 'Auto' means 'self', and 'phagy' means 'eating' or 'devouring'. So autophagy means 'self-eating'. That might sound like some kind of horrible disease, but it is actually a vital process that keeps us healthy. You see, when cells 'eat themselves', they don't just randomly gobble up stuff. Autophagy is used to specifically break down damaged cellular components, whether they are individual molecules or entire cellular 'organs' – what is called organelles.

You can consider autophagy as the cell's garbage collection system. The cell uses small bubble-like structures (like garbage bags) to engulf damaged molecules or cellular components. Then it transports the 'garbage bags' to special organelles called lysosomes, which are like recycling stations. Lysosomes contain various enzymes that break down the cellular garbage into its building blocks. And afterwards, these building blocks can be released and reused for making new molecules.

This garbage/recycling system – and others like it – actually unites *everything* we have discussed so far. For one, autophagy is what awaits us at the bottom of our rabbit hole. We started at growth hormone being released from the pituitary gland. Upon reaching the liver, we learned that growth hormone promotes production of IGF-1. And when IGF-1 binds to cell receptors, it activates the protein complex mTOR. Now, to be fair, mTOR does *a lot* of things, many of which impact health. But the thing that is most obviously tied to ageing is that mTOR controls the cellular garbage collection system. Specifically, when mTOR is active, it *blocks* autophagy. And in turn, all the growth-promoting signals that activate mTOR do the same thing. So when rapamycin blocks mTOR, it essentially blocks the blocker, cancelling it out. This might sound a little confusing, but the bottom line is that blocking growth signals ends up *activating* autophagy. As a result, rapamycin only prolongs the life of laboratory organisms as long as autophagy is functional. If autophagy is broken, rapamycin stops working. So it really does seem like we have reached the end of this whole thing.

Besides all the stuff relating to growth, though, autophagy is also a vital part of hormesis. It's important to remember that while damage can strengthen us in the long run, it is not the actual damage that is beneficial. For instance, right after you go for a run, you are weaker than you were before. And free radicals – the rampaging bull – *are* harmful. The reason they can make us stronger over time, is that our cells have the ability to repair and subsequently improve. The first step is exactly what autophagy does: collecting and disposing of damaged molecules. So autophagy is a key part of hormesis, too. If the cellular garbage collection system doesn't function optimally, various forms of hormesis stop extending the lifespan of laboratory organisms.

Unfortunately, despite its importance to lifespan, autophagy slowly declines with age. For reasons not entirely understood, our cellular garbage collectors get lazy and bad at their job over time. This is one of the reasons cells tend to accumulate old and damaged proteins as they age. It was once believed old cells filled up with 'cellular junk' like this because they were more sensitive to damage than young cells. But actually, it's just as important that old cells are simply bad at *removing* junk, making it accumulate. So should you and I try to increase autophagy in our cells? Studies in mice suggest so. When scientists artificially increase autophagy activity in mice, the mice get stronger and leaner, and ultimately, they also live longer. On the other hand, if autophagy is inhibited in mice, damaged molecules quickly accumulate, and the mice become weak and sickly.

(Scientists cannot make mice that completely lack autophagy, because this would prove lethal before the mice are even born.)

The fighting naked mole-rat

Naked mole-rats are much better than their close relatives, mice, at surviving stressors such as DNA-damaging chemicals, heavy metals or extreme heat. At the same time, the cells of naked mole-rats have considerably more autophagy activity than the cells of mice. Naked mole-rats also have higher activity in another cellular waste disposal system – the proteasome system – which specifically deals with breaking down damaged proteins. Similarly, other small yet long-lived mammals, bats, *upregulate* autophagy as they age. The increased activity among the cellular garbage collectors could be the reason bats and naked mole-rats live so much longer than other mammals of the same size.

When summer arrives, the population of my home town, Copenhagen, seems to triple. If you also live somewhere with dark and cold winters, you probably recognise the allure of the summer sun. Most of us enjoy some sunbathing, and some turn summers into a months-long quest for the perfect tan.

What actually happens when you sunbathe is that your skin is exposed to UV radiation and gets damaged by it. This initiates a cascade of signals inside your cells, which eventually makes them produce the pigment melanin to protect themselves.

Sunbathing is no problem in small doses – it might even be hormetic – but if you overdo it, your risk of skin cancer and wrinkles increases dramatically. Wouldn't it be a lot easier if we didn't have to risk skin cancer (and turning into a raisin) to get a tan? A clever way to do this would be to find another way to initiate the signal cascade normally induced by UV-damage. That is, fake the signal that eventually makes us produce melanin. If done right, your cells wouldn't be able to tell the difference. They would just see the message: 'Make more melanin,' and they'd comply. Some scientists have actually already proven this strategy in the lab. They have succeeded in using a special molecule to kick-start melanin production in both mice and human skin samples. So maybe future sunscreen will not just be used to protect you from the sun – it might also be what makes you tan without the need to lie on a sunbed for hours.

You can imagine a similar strategy for autophagy. Right now, our best bet for activating autophagy is either blocking various growth signals or using hormesis. Both options come with potential side effects. And besides, despite all these efforts, your cellular garbage collectors will still get lazy as you age. What we need is another way to deliver the message 'go clean up'.

Perhaps we could even find ways to stimulate autophagy more strongly in old age than we can at present.

I'm happy to report that the first candidate for an autophagy booster has already been found, though we are still awaiting human trials. This compound reliably increases autophagy in cells, and when scientists add it to the drinking water of mice, they live longer than normal – even if the treatment starts later in life. The molecule in question is called spermidine. You can probably guess where it was originally discovered, but don't worry. There are other sources of spermidine.

First, your cells actually produce spermidine and similar compounds themselves. However, our own spermidine production tends to decrease with age, just like autophagy does. And right now, we don't know of any reliable way to reverse this.

Second, spermidine is also produced by some species of gut bacteria. However, once again, we don't know how to influence this process. Other gut bacteria *break down* spermidine, and the whole thing is too complicated to mess with at present.

Fortunately, the third option – diet – is easier to influence. Spermidine is found in many foods, and studies even show that a higher spermidine intake is associated with a lower risk of death. If you want to increase your spermidine intake, the best bet is wheatgerm. Actually, spermidine cannot be made into a supplement, so even if you do see spermidine 'supplements', they will just be wheatgerm with extra spermidine content. Besides that, other spermidine-containing foods include soy beans, certain mushrooms, sunflower seeds, corn and cauliflower. If you're more adventurous, you can also try eel liver, adzuki beans or durian fruit.

Chapter 9
Infamous High School Biology

Over a billion years ago, somewhere in a random hot puddle, a bacterium was engulfed by a cell that is an early ancestor to all of us. Exactly how it happened, we don't know. Maybe the cell meant for the bacterium to be a simple meal. Or maybe the aggressor was the bacterium; a parasite looking for a new home. Whatever happened, the bacterium ended up inside the cell and it has stuck around for a long time. In fact, its descendants are still a part of you and me today.

You see, while the bacterium and ancestor cell were two different species, today they are one. Through millions of years of evolution, the two have merged with each other and can no longer be separated.

We call the descendants of this bacterium 'mitochondria', and they are a vital part of our cells. If we were to look inside your cells right now, we would find anything from a few to several thousand mitochondria. These mitochondria still bear resemblance to their bacterial past: they are shaped and structured like bacteria, and even still act a little bit like bacteria. For instance, your mitochondria make more mito-chondria in the same way as bacteria make more bacteria: by dividing. That said, your mitochondria are not something separate from you. They are closely integrated with the rest of the cell as an organelle (a cellular organ). And your mito-chondria are not viable on their own anymore, either. They can only exist as part of your cells. Through millions of years of evolution, the vast majority of mitochondrial DNA has been moved to the nucleus of the cell with the rest of your genetic blueprint. Only a tiny bit remains in the mitochon-dria themselves as a reminder of their independent heritage.

★ ★ ★

You might already know the role of mitochondria thanks to that most infamous quote of high school biology: *Mito-chondria are the powerhouse of the cell.* While many people are annoyed they have to learn this, it actually makes mitochon-dria one of the most important organelles in your cells. They are responsible for the last part of the cellular task that makes everything else possible: harvesting energy from the food you eat. As a result, the amount of mitochondria in cells varies by function. Your muscle cells, especially heart muscle cells, have a lot of mitochondria because they use a lot of energy. Other cell types, such as skin cells, are mostly tasked with sitting around, and thus they have few mitochondria.

Power plants really are the best analogy for mitochondria and you want all the properties from your mitochondria that you'd want from your local power plant: reliability, safety and minimal impact on the environment. Evolution has made sure your mitochondria are highly optimised to fulfil this job. However, as with most other things in our cells, ageing tends to ruin the system. As we age, we lose mitochondria, and those that remain tend to become dysfunctional. You can think of it as going from lots of shiny new power plants to a few old and worn-out ones.

This decline in mitochondrial function spells trouble, as energy is necessary for everything the cell does. Studies show that dysfunctional mitochondria promote ageing in laboratory organisms, and we see the effect of their dysfunction in humans too. For instance, loss of mitochondria is one of the reasons our muscles tend to get weaker with age. So, what can we do to keep the cellular power plants humming?

The answer to that question is a list of our old acquaintances. Like many other biological systems, mitochondria experience hormesis. The main way to beneficially challenge these organelles is by increasing your energy needs, especially acutely. Two things come to mind. First, exercise, especially exercise with a high intensity. And second, cold exposure, for instance in the form of winter swimming.

One of the ways mitochondria respond to being challenged is through something called 'mitochondrial biogenesis'. This just means mitochondria dividing to make more of themselves. That's good, because it increases the capacity of the cells, and it also counteracts the loss of mitochondria that normally happens during ageing. In fact, it seems you can pretty much entirely cancel out the age-related loss of mitochondria if you exercise sufficiently.

Another response to mitochondrial hormesis is autophagy, or 'mitophagy', as some call it when related to mitochondria. This process ensures that old and dysfunctional cellular power plants are regularly removed. In fact, the removal of damaged mitochondria is one of the most important roles played by autophagy. As a result, autophagy boosters like spermidine particularly impact mitochondria. When researchers give mice spermidine to extend their lives, it turns out the most important effect is mediated through mitophagy, in particular the removal of dysfunctional cellular power plants in heart muscle cells. Treatment with spermidine improves heart health in the mice and ensures a clean energy supply. This is pretty important, as we would prefer for the heart to keep beating. (In fact, it is not just the spermidine mice that have healthier hearts. We also know that, among humans, a higher spermidine intake in the diet is associated with a lower risk of cardiovascular disease.)

Scientists have also identified another compound, called urolithin A, which can increase mitophagy. When researchers give urolithin A to elderly, non-active people, there's an increase in mitophagy in their muscles. The same thing happens in mice, improving their endurance as a result. And it turns out urolithin A doesn't just improve mitophagy: it also stimulates mitochondria to divide, which is the same thing that happens after exercise.

Unfortunately, urolithin A doesn't occur naturally in food. Or at least, no one has found it yet. However, precursors to the urolithin A molecule are found in pomegranates, walnuts and raspberries in the form of polyphenols called ellagitannins. And it turns out some gut bacteria can convert ellagitannins into urolithin A. Not everyone has these species in their gut, though, but generally speaking, eating more pomegranates, walnuts and raspberries can never be a bad thing.

Nature is fond of recycling

While the main role of your mitochondria is as the powerhouse of the cell, nature is fond of recycling. For whatever reason, mitochondria have other functions that don't relate much to their power plant job. One example is that the trigger for cellular suicide – apoptosis – sits on the mitochondria. And in addition, mitochondria are also involved in our immune system – both in killing enemies and in signalling pathways that control the whole thing.

Chapter 10

Adventures in Immortality

In the winter of 1951, a thirty-one-year-old woman named Henrietta Lacks was admitted to Johns Hopkins Hospital in Baltimore, Maryland. Lacks was complaining of feeling a 'knot' on her cervix and believed she might be pregnant again. But instead, doctors found a visible lesion. She had cancer. Through 1951, the cancer metastasised and spread all over Lacks' body, ultimately killing her later that year.

Before the death of Henrietta Lacks, doctors had studied cells from her cervical biopsy in culture in the laboratory. Normally, this is hard. Human cells are not fond of growing in culture and tend to die quickly outside the body. But the cancer cells of Henrietta Lacks seemed to thrive just fine. Doctors were baffled as they watched the cells dutifully divide, day after day.

When Henrietta Lacks passed away, her cell sample was still very much alive in the laboratory. And this is where the story gets murky. As the cells of Henrietta Lacks were the first culturable human cell line that was a big deal scientifically. The scientists involved started eagerly sharing the cells with other scientists, but they never consulted Henrietta Lacks or her family. I will let you be the judge of the morals here; Johns Hopkins issued an apology over 50 years later.

The point is that the cells of Henrietta Lacks live on to this day. The cell line, called HeLa, is immortal, and the free sharing of cells means that it is used all over the world today. Just a few years after the death of Henrietta Lacks, it was used by Jonas Salk to develop the first vaccine against polio. And since then, HeLa cells have been used millions of times in cancer research, virology and basic biomedical science.

★ ★ ★

At the end of a shoelace, there's a piece of plastic or metal that ensures the lace doesn't fray. I bet you never wondered what those things are called. They're aglets. That might sound like a completely irrelevant fact in a book about ageing research, but your cells actually face a similar problem to that dealt with by shoelace manufacturers. You see, inside your cells, your DNA is contained in long thread-like structures called chromosomes. And the ends of these chromosomes can get damaged or frayed, just like the tips of shoelaces. Your cells solve the problem with something called telomeres, which are like genetic shoelace aglets. Telomeres are made from the same building blocks as the rest of your DNA – nucleotides – but the difference is that telomeres don't contain any important information. They have no genes, and are just made up of the same sequence repeated again and again. That's clever, because it means our cells can lose some telomere and be alright. At least in the short term. In the long term, our telomeres are actually a cornerstone in determining the lifespan of our cells.

We once thought cells were immortal, even though organisms as a whole age and die. But then a scientist named Leonard Hayflick proved that normal human cells will die after they have divided a set number of times. This phenomenon is now called 'Hayflick's limit' and it is caused by our telomeres. When we're born, our telomeres consist of approximately 11,000 nucleotides. But every time our cells divide, the telomeres get a little bit shorter. That's fine, until they become so short that our useful DNA becomes jeopardised. Before this can happen, the cell pulls the emergency brake and stops dividing.

In this way, the shortening of telomeres is what makes cells mortal. Even if we somehow enabled cells to continue dividing after they reach Hayflick's limit, cells would eventually lose the telomeres entirely. That would expose DNA to damage and the cell would die anyway.

However, maybe you can think of at least one possible solution. What if we just elongated the telomeres to cancel out the loss? That's actually what some cells do. We have an enzyme called telomerase, which is what makes our telomeres in the first place. You can think of telomerase as a little molecular machine that goes to the end of chromosomes and elongates the telomeres. Cells mostly use telomerase during development when we grow from a single cell to billions in a short time. That requires a lot of cellular divisions, and telomerase makes sure we don't run out of telomeres before life even gets started. Soon after development is finished, though, the vast majority of our cells turn off the telomerase gene and become mortal.

★ ★ ★

Telomerase is the reason the cancer cells of Henrietta Lacks became immortal. Lacks' cancer was caused by the virus HPV-18 (Human Papillomavirus 18), which causes the majority of cervical cancers in the world. In the process of infecting Lacks, the virus turned on the gene that makes telomerase.

That means the virus gave the cells an ability to continuously elongate their telomeres and thus divide again and again without ever running out. That's pretty helpful for a cancer, and it's also what keeps the HeLa cells immortal to this day. If scientists block the telomerase enzyme in the HeLa cells, they lose their immortality and die after a set number of divisions, just like their pre-cancerous ancestors.

Think about that for a moment. We actually know how to make cells immortal. And you and I consist of lots of cells – 37 trillion, to be exact. However, is making cells immortal the same as making the organism immortal? If it is, the way to prolong life is to keep our telomeres from becoming short. Researchers have investigated this approach by breeding mice that are born with abnormally long telomeres. Not only are these mice leaner than normal mice, they also have healthier metabolisms, age better – and, ultimately, live longer.

We also have suggestive evidence from humans. People born with mutations that cause rapid shortening of the telomeres age prematurely. And even within the normal variation, telomeres are associated with ageing. As with all other traits, there are differences in telomere-related characteristics between individuals. Some people have longer telomeres than others, and some people lose telomeres more slowly throughout life. In a Danish study of 65,000 people, those with shorter telomeres had a higher mortality rate and a higher rate of age-related diseases, such as cardiovascular diseases and Alzheimer's.

So, should we try to elongate our telomeres? Scientists haven't tried this officially – but someone outside the normal bounds of academia has.

★ ★ ★

In 2015, an American woman travelled to Colombia hoping to launch a life-extension revolution. Liz Parrish, as she is called, is neither a mad scientist nor a rich weirdo. In many ways, she is your average suburban mum.

While working on stem cell advocacy, Parrish learned about the powers of telomerase. Scientists showed her how mice with long telomeres will be bouncing around full of youthful energy while similarly aged normal mice will sit in the corner, old and frail.

Parrish dreamed of transferring this magic to humans, but learned that it would be hard. Scientists have tried making drugs that turn on the telomerase enzyme, but it has proven very difficult. Instead, Parrish opted to use something called gene therapy. This is a newer medical invention where scientists add an extra gene to a person's cells, a bit like adding a spare part. In this case, the genetic spare part would be an extra (and active) telomerase gene.

Liz Parrish didn't travel to Colombia because Colombians especially need to have their telomeres elongated. Instead, she left her home country to get away from the Food and Drug Administration. Parrish wanted to use herself as the first test person, but the United States, and most other developed countries, severely restricts the type of medical procedures you're allowed to carry out – even if it's just to your own body. Injecting a gene therapy you came up with yourself would never fly.

And so, Parrish flew instead. In Colombia, she found a clinic that was willing to help her out. First, scientific collaborators measured Parrish's telomeres so that the efficacy of the treatment could be determined. They found that she actually had significantly shorter telomeres than expected for a woman her age. Not the worst test person.

Then, Parrish received her gene therapy injections, and after a bit of monitoring for acute side effects, she went back to her home country. The following year, it was time for the results, and once again, Parrish's scientific collaborators measured the length of her telomeres. The results were positive. It seems Liz Parrish is the first person ever to successfully elongate her telomeres.

★ ★ ★

Liz Parrish's self-experiment caused an uproar in the scientific community. On one side, proponents argued that the self-experiment would provide valuable data for the rest of us. On the other side, critics considered the whole ordeal dangerous – reckless, even – and feared social contagion. Parrish herself has defended her position and has been quoted as saying: 'To get US government approval to bring gene therapies to you . . . I would have to go raise almost a billion dollars. It would take about fifteen years of testing. And when I'm looking out there, I'm seeing people who don't want to wait fifteen years.'

However, let's take a step back. It's true that we could argue about whether or not a self-experiment like this is safe. But the most important question is whether it would be worthwhile even *if* it worked. Think about it: I told you all our cells have the gene for telomerase. But early in life, they turn it off and keep it like that. If the secret to a long life is telomerase, why wouldn't our cells just turn the enzyme back on and use it?

The reason turns out to be an ugly trade-off. Maybe you can guess it from the story of Henrietta Lacks. It is true that telomerase can make cells immortal. But that's exactly what the cells of Henrietta Lacks became – and how did that turn out for her? The problem is that the telomerase gene is essential in the development of cancer. Eighty to ninety per cent of all human cancers find some kind of way to turn on the telomerase gene. Even the ones that don't do this usually find another way to elongate their telomeres. They have to. Without continuous elongation of the telomeres, the cancer cells would eventually die, just like normal cells.

To be fair, advocates for telomere extension, such as Parrish, don't favour immortalising one's cells. They hope to turn on telomerase briefly – just enough to slightly elongate the telomeres, but not enough to make cells cancerous. It's not actually clear whether those things can be separated, though. Studies show that people who have longer-than-average telomeres are at a higher risk of getting cancer. So it seems that messing with telomeres is a dangerous project at best. As our ability to fight cancer keeps improving, it might someday become worth it to take the bet. But until then, I'd stay away. Nature has probably already considered the ageing/cancer trade-off and set telomere length accordingly.

Besides, there are also other problems with telomere research: mainly that most studies use mice as their model organism. Mice are often a good way to model humans, taking cost and difficulty into account, but they're not a good model organism when it comes to telomeres. Telomere biology in mice is very different than it is in us; mice have active telomerase in all their cells and are also born with much longer telomeres than we are. If telomeres were the only source of youth, mice would live substantially longer than us. But they don't – mice struggle to live even a few years while succumbing to cancer at high rates. On to the next one.

Telomeres in space

In 2016, American astronaut Scott Kelly came back from what was then the longest stay for an American aboard the International Space Station. Back on Earth, he was met by his loved ones, including his identical twin brother, Mark Kelly, who is also an astronaut. NASA examined both twins before, during and after the journey to learn about the physical effects of long stays in space. They found that spacefaring Scott underwent many physiological changes that earthbound Mark didn't. One of them was that Scott's telomeres got *longer* while he was in space. But once he was back on Earth, they quickly shortened again, and actually ended up shorter than they were before the trip.

Maybe the Fountain of Youth is a one-way ticket to space . . .

Chapter 11
Zombie Cells and How to Get Rid of Them

In the tombs of ancient Greece, skeletons are often weighed down with stones and other heavy objects, as though to prevent the dead from resurrecting. And even further back, in ancient Mesopotamia, there are stories like the one about the goddess Ishtar, who threatens, 'I will let the dead rise and eat the living.' Today, we still have these kinds of horror stories about the living dead – zombies – and they have made it into this book as well. The zombies we're going to encounter, though, are different from the Hollywood ones. Our zombies are zombie *cells*.

★ ★ ★

Normally, cells anxiously monitor their own condition. If they sense something is wrong, they will kill themselves in cellular suicide – what's called apoptosis. This is why human cells are hard to grow in the laboratory. When the cells are removed from the body, they notice that something is off and promptly kill themselves. This level of paranoia might seem drastic, but as always, there's an evolutionary reason your cells behave like this. Cellular suicide is a mechanism to prevent cancer and fight infections. If one of your cells suspects it's turning cancerous or has been infected with a virus, it selflessly sacrifices itself to save the rest of your body. That might sound heroic, but it is actually a completely normal part of how your body works. In fact, while you've been reading this paragraph alone, a few million of your cells have killed themselves. Yes, millions. You lose between 50 and 70 *billion* cells to apoptosis every day. That is a mindbogglingly large number, but it's actually just a tiny fraction of your cells, and your body can easily replace them.

In some cases, damaged cells don't outright kill themselves, but instead enter a state called cellular senescence. This is what we call zombie cells. Senescence was first described by Leonard Hayflick as the result of reaching Hayflick's limit. That is, cells can end up as zombie cells when they run out of telomeres. But there are plenty of other ways, too. In general, all the types of damage that can lead a cell to cellular suicide can also make it become a zombie cell instead.

When a cell turns into a zombie cell, it stops most of its normal activity, including ceasing to divide. But instead of dying, which would be an obvious next step, the cell sticks around. And on top of that, it starts spewing out a cocktail of damaging molecules into its surroundings. It's not a long stretch to imagine cells like that could promote ageing. So scientists from the Mayo Clinic in Minnesota set out to investigate how zombie cells affect the lifespan of biological organisms. In one study, the scientist isolated zombie cells from old mice and transplanted them into young, healthy mice. The young mice started out full of vigour but it took just a single dose of zombie cells to slow them down. Curiously, the mice remained weak, even six months after the transplantation, when the original zombie cells were long gone. The reason turns out to be that zombie cells – in true zombie fashion – spread their condition to other cells. The molecules they spew out in their surroundings can make normal, healthy cells become zombie cells as well – even cells that are located in totally different areas of the body. As a result, the mice of the experiment never recovered from the zombie cell transplantation. They ended up dying earlier than normal mice, and the more zombie cells were transplanted, the worse they fared.

What happened to these poor mice is actually somewhat similar to what happens during normal ageing. We're not suddenly injected with zombie cells, but as we grow old, zombie cells tend to accumulate in the body. An old person has many more zombie cells than a young person. And given that zombie cells clearly have a negative effect, perhaps it would be beneficial to get rid of them outright? Researchers – again from the Mayo Clinic – have tested this using some ingenious genetic engineering. In short, the researchers made mice with cells containing a special genetic construct. You can imagine the construct as a little bomb that would only be active in zombie cells, and which the researchers could trigger on command using a special trigger molecule. Upon administering this molecule to the mice, the 'cellular bomb' would go off in zombie cells and kill them.

The researchers divided their genetically engineered mice into two groups to test the effect of removing zombie cells. The first group was left alone while the researchers triggered the cellular bomb twice-weekly in the other group. It was necessary to kill the zombie cells continuously like this because zombie cells appear throughout life. By targeting them again and again, the scientists made sure their mice remained zombie-free. As expected, getting rid of the zombie cells proved a boon for the mice. The scientists noted that the zombie-free mice looked significantly healthier and more energetic than their zombie-plagued peers. And ultimately, the zombie-free mice also lived around twenty-five per cent longer than the control mice.

★ ★ ★

So, should you and I be looking for a way to get rid of our own zombie cells? It is important to note that cellular senescence is not always a damaging phenomenon. Zombie cells actually play an important role in both our development and in wound healing, which should not be disrupted. However, the mice studies from above pretty clearly implicate zombie cells in age-ing, and there's even signs zombie cells help promote several age-related diseases. It seems cellular senescence is a helpful mechanism in youth but gets derailed over time.

The immune system somehow plays a role here. Normally, immune cells can eat and remove the zombie cells. In fact, the damaging molecules spewed out by zombie cells are partly used to attract immune cells. But in old age, the zombie cells call in vain. Ageing robs us of immune cells, and those that are still around are often occupied elsewhere.

That means we will have to find another way to rid ourselves of the zombie cells. You and I don't have any 'cellular bomb' encoded in our genes, so we will have to come up with something else. There are two options. We could try to 'rescue' the zombie cells, turning them back into normal, healthy cells. Or we could try to kill the zombies.

Option two sounds more fun, and it seems cellular senescence researchers agree. At least, zombie killing is by far the most researched option. Unfortunately, however, killing zombie cells is not as easy as killing zombies in the movies. The main obstacle is that zombie cells don't all hang out together. They're spread out throughout the body and are always in the minority, even in old age. As a result, you have to be very accurate when targeting zombie cells. Even slight inaccuracy would mean you end up killing many more normal cells than zombie cells. That would be a net negative.

Despite the difficulty, scientists *have* managed to find drug candidates that target zombie cells specifically. These drugs are called 'senolytics', and most of them kill by forcing the zombie cells into cellular suicide. As we've discussed, this is the fate most zombie cells were destined for anyway before they became zombie cells instead. The zombie cells inhibit the cellular suicide response, but senolytic compounds can force their hands.

The senolytics found so far include many compounds derived from plants. So, once again, I'm reminding you to eat your fruit and vegetables. One example of a senolytic molecule is a flavonoid called fisetin, which is found in strawberries and apples. Adding extra fisetin to the chow of old mice improves their lifespan, even when started late in life. The study in question used much higher concentrations of fisetin than you'd realistically get from your food, though. If you wanted an equivalent amount, you'd have to eat a few kilos of strawberries. Now you have the excuse.

Other examples of zombie-killing compounds that can extend the life of mice include the flavonoid procyanidin C1, which is found in grapes and also fisetin's close cousin, quercetin, which is found in onions and cabbage. Quercetin is especially well-researched in combination with the drug dasatinib. This combination is much more powerful than quercetin alone. Now, dasatinib is a leukaemia drug, so not something you'd eat on a normal day. But the combination of dasatinib and quercetin is currently being investigated in humans in several clinical trials. They're a good candidate for a future pharmaceutical solution to zombie cells, but a leukaemia drug is obviously not something to play around with. In general, even though some of the zombie-killing compounds can be found as supplements, caution is warranted. At high concentrations, these molecules are toxic to normal cells too. Anyone experimenting with them should really know what they are doing.

The best approach to fighting our zombie cells is to cross our fingers and watch the clinical trials. There's actually already been a success story: an experimental senolytic drug has been used to safely improve two age-related eye conditions. Given the tons of money involved and many different trials, it's possible a senolytic will be the first real anti-ageing drug approved by medical authorities. In the meantime, there's a bunch of – admittedly less effective – ways of combating zombie cells.

First, viral infections can turn cells into zombie cells. And interestingly, some viruses, like influenza type A, can be fought using senolytic compounds like quercetin.

Second, there's the immune angle. A healthy immune system would probably be able to take care of the zombie cell problem all on its own.

Third, it is interesting to note that most zombie-killing compounds are flavonoids from plants. Sure, to get the amounts used in these studies, you'd have to eat like an elephant. But there are lots of plant compounds similar to these. Who knows if they have a synergistic effect together.

And finally, while we've established it's more fun to kill the zombie cells, there's also exciting research taking place that aims to reverse the condition. Several studies have shown that the circadian rhythm hormone melatonin can help bring zombie cells back to a healthy state. Melatonin is not the 'sleep hormone' as it is sometimes described, but optimising sleep and having a consistent wake/sleep schedule is a good idea.

Chapter 12
Winding the Biological Clock

Imagine that you're a scientist working on a new drug to combat ageing. You start moving up the ladder of laboratory organisms. It works in yeast. Then in *C. elegans*. Then in fruit flies. And, finally, in mice too. You're very excited. After some speculation, you decide to take the leap and bet on this drug. Years go by with safety tests, fundraising, dosage experiments and a lot of bureaucracy. But eventually, you're ready to answer the big question: will your new drug work in humans? You sit down to plan the trial. How are you going to find out? Are you going to give your drug to a bunch of middle-aged people? Then you'll have to wait for decades to find out if they lived longer than usual. Instead, you could give your drug to people who are *already* old. But even this trial will take many years – and by using old people, you're giving your drug less time to work. You could end up in a situation where the trial fails but is still suggestive of some benefit. Then you either have to give up, or revert to the original plan: giving your drug to middle-aged people while waiting the rest of your career to see what happens.

As you might imagine, this 'waiting dilemma' is extremely annoying to biomedical scientists. It's one of the main obstacles for anyone trying to develop preventative medicine. If you want to prevent, say, dementia or cancer, it will take years before you know if a potential drug works. Only then can you adjust your approach accordingly. And mind you, even making it to the point where you *can* test a drug takes many years and costs millions of dollars. So it is really no surprise that progress in medicine tends to be slower than in many other areas of science and technology.

The huge time investment required for drug development is why researchers are excited by what are called biomarkers. A biomarker is a surrogate indicator for some important biological outcome. It's something you can easily measure that helps tell you about a particular biological state. For instance, during a fever, your temperature rises. That means we can use body temperature as a biomarker for fever intensity. If we give you a new drug, and your body temperature starts falling, it might be because the drug is treating whatever is causing your fever.

You can imagine another biomarker that, instead of 'tracking' the progression of a fever, tracks biological age. That is, it describes how old you are *biologically* as opposed to the number of candles on your birthday cake. In more morbid words, a biomarker for biological age would accurately describe how close you are to death. We're well aware that two people who might be the same age *chronologically* can have bodies in wildly different physical conditions. Some seventy-year-olds are busy running marathons, while others are struggling to walk to the corner shop. In this case, the first person might be fifty-five biologically, while the other person is eighty-five biologically.

So, if you had a biological clock, your drug-development efforts would be much easier. At the start of your trial, you'd get baseline measurements. Then, you'd make two groups with similar characteristics and give the subjects in one group your drug.

Now, instead of waiting for years until people die, you'd occasionally measure their biological ages. If your drug really works, it will slow down the biological ageing of those receiving it. That means they would be biologically younger at later measurements than the control group, who would continue to age normally. And in that way, you'd save yourself a whole lot of time.

★ ★ ★

Among the first 'biological clocks' proposed were telomeres. At first glance, they seem a good match. As you might remember, our telomeres gradually get shorter throughout our lives, and shorter telomeres tend to correlate with an earlier death. For this reason, many studies *do* use telomeres as a biological clock, and they are better than nothing. However, telomere-shortening is not as reliable a biological clock as we might wish. Yes, on average, people with shorter telomeres tend to die younger but the correlation is far from perfect. And if we zoom out, away from just humans, the picture gets murkier still. Mice, as we've seen, have longer telomeres than humans, yet live much shorter lives. And scientists have even found a seabird, Leach's storm petrel, that has telomeres that get *longer* as it ages (interestingly, this bird also has a long lifespan for its size). Clearly, telomeres don't reflect the whole phenomenon we call ageing.

In 2013, the German-American scientist Steve Horvath presented a new biological clock that beats telomere-shortening, along with pretty much everything else we have. This new biological clock is often called 'the epigenetic clock', and the way it works is a little complicated. But let's give it a shot.

As the name implies, the epigenetic clock is based on something called epigenetics. You can think of epigenetics as a control system inside your cells. Remember, all your cells (except red blood cells) have all of your DNA – the entire genetic recipe for making you. But for the most part, your cells only need a tiny fraction of the recipe at any given time. Your muscle cells need to use genes that help make muscle fibres, but they don't need the genes that make dental enamel or taste receptors. Cells that make your teeth, on the other hand, *do* need the genes for making dental enamel but not the genes for making muscle fibres. And besides, even *if* a cell needs a specific gene, it doesn't necessarily need it all the time.

The solution to this is a control system that can manage which genes are used in the cell at any given time. When the cell needs a gene, it can turn it on. When it doesn't, it can shut it down.

Part of this control system is epigenetics: reversible chemical changes to your DNA. You can imagine the cell putting different tags on genes – 'turn on', 'turn on soon', 'switch off temporarily', 'switch off permanently', and so on. It's pretty ingenious, actually. In this way, our cells can use the same genetic recipe to make brain cells, immune cells, cells in your pinkie and everything in between.

Epigenetics are especially useful during development, when we grow from a tiny ball of cells to an infant, a child and later an adult. Some genes are only needed during early development, some are needed to become a certain type of cell, and some are useful for growing up and becoming a mature adult. However, at that point, we would then expect our epigenetics to stay relatively set. After all, once you've become an adult, the programme has successfully run to completion. But surprisingly, epigenetic changes keep happening, even later in life. Scientists used to believe this was simply due to cellular machinery getting faulty with age. They imagined cells slowly losing control and ending up putting essentially random tags on genes. To support this, most of the age-related epigenetic changes are loss of the ability to turn genes off effectively. This becomes a hazard when genes involved in growth are activated even though we finished growing long ago, because this growth promotion can stimulate the growth of cancers.

Despite this neat story, Steve Horvath has proved that epigenetic changes later in life are not random after all. They keep following a specific pattern, almost as if the developmental programme continues. Programmed ageing? In order to remain sane, scientists have resolved to call this pattern 'quasi-programmed'. Whatever the reason, though, the predictability of epigenetic changes can be used to determine the biological age of a cell. The epigenetic clock uses a particular epigenetic 'tag' called methylation which is used to turn genes off. Scientists measure the amount of methylation in specific genetic places and because the age-related changes follow a pattern, they can use statistics to determine biological age with high accuracy. For instance, people whose epigenetic age is higher than their actual age are at greater risk of dying early. They also have a greater risk of getting age-related diseases, such as cardiovascular disease, cancer and Alzheimer's. And they even *seem* older, performing worse on cognitive tests and being physically weaker. On the other hand, centenarians reliably turn out to be younger biologically than their actual age, which is probably why they are still alive: their actual age might be 106, while the biological state of their body is much younger than that.

In fact, newer versions of the epigenetic clock work so well that they can even be used in other species. First, this was done in chimpanzees, but now there are epigenetic clocks that work for all other mammals, too. That suggests these clocks measure something very fundamental about the ageing process.

★ ★ ★

Since their creation, researchers have been busy using epigenetic clocks to peek into all sorts of interesting aspects of ageing. One example is the way ageing works in different parts of the body. You see, chronologically, all your cells and tissues are the same age. Some cell types might have short *individual* lifespans, but these cells are recently descended from stem cells – the cells that make other cells. And in the end, all your cells descend from the first cell that was uniquely you, the fertilised egg. The epigenetic clock corroborates this, as all cells have roughly the same biological age. This means you can use all sorts of different cell types from the same person – brain cells, liver cells, skin cells – and the epigenetic clock will show the same biological age. However, there *are* a few exceptions, and these tell us some fascinating things about ageing. Most notably, women's breast tissue tends to be biologically older than any other tissue studied. This is thought-provoking, because breast cancer is the most common cancer in women, costing millions of lives each year. We're all aware that breast cancer is a big menace, because there are so many support groups and fundraisers for it. But I'm not sure someone completely naive would have guessed one of the most common cancers to be in the breasts. Why there and not one of the dozen other organs? If the reason is that breast tissue ages more rapidly, that at least gives a little bit of an explanation. In fact, premature cellular ageing must be involved: studies show that the higher the epigenetic age of a woman's breast tissue compared to her actual age, the greater her risk of breast cancer. Of course, this only raises the next big question: why does breast tissue tend to age more rapidly? We don't really know. But once we find the answer, we might be able to use it in the development of breast cancer therapies and preventative medicine. And in the process, we might also learn some things about cellular ageing that can be broadly applicable.

At the other end of the spectrum, there's also a specific tissue that tends to age more *slowly* than the rest of the body. The part of the brain called the cerebellum usually has the lowest epigenetic age in a person. The cerebellum is not a part of the body non-scientists hear that much about. Perhaps one reason is that not much stuff tends to go wrong here – at least, the cerebellum is far less afflicted by age-related diseases than the rest of the brain. Again, we don't really know why, but maybe studies of ageing in the cerebellum can help us learn how to slow down ageing in the rest of the brain, and decrease the risk of neurodegenerative diseases.

The female advantage

Women tend to live longer than men, and they also have lower epigenetic ages on average. In fact, this is already evident by the age of two. The female advantage is especially evident before menopause. Until then, women seem partially protected against age-related diseases. And only after menopause does the female risk profile slowly start to converge with the male one. Interestingly, women who go through menopause later than average also tend to live longer than average. And the epigenetic clock gives us an idea why. Women who have their ovaries removed surgically – and thus enter menopause artificially early – have higher biological ages than expected. On the other hand,

---

women who delay menopause using hormone therapy have lower biological ages than expected.

Unfortunately, hormone therapy increases the risk of breast cancer, so this area is a bit like the telomeres. If only we had better cancer therapies, we might have a highly beneficial anti-ageing therapy.

You started your life as a single cell – the result of a fusion between the egg cell provided by your mother and the sperm cell provided by your father. After the fusion, the fertilised egg quickly began to divide, forming a little ball of cells. All these early cells were what scientists called 'pluripotent', which means they were cells retaining the ability to morph into any of the more than 200 cell types that make up your body today. However, as you developed, your cells continuously special-ised, closing off options as they went. You can imagine it like climbing up a big tree. At the trunk, the cell retains the ability to climb out on any branch that it wants. Then, at one point, the cell chooses a major branch, and this limits the cell types it can later become. Continuing up the tree, options are limited by each further choice until the cell ends up on a particular branch: the 'finished product', such as brain cells, muscle cells or skin cells. This is what's called terminally differentiated cells.

Scientists once thought that this climb was a one-way thing: that once a cell had committed to a particular fate, there was no way to reverse the decision. But then Japanese scientist Shinya Yamanaka proved everyone wrong (and later won the Nobel Prize in Medicine in 2012). Yamanaka showed that terminally differentiated cells can be made *back* into pluripotent cells.

That is, we could take one of your skin cells and coax it into crawling all the way back to the trunk of our hypothetical tree. Yamanaka and his research group reset development this way by using four proteins, which are now called 'the Yamanaka factors'. Once these are activated in the cell, 'de-development' takes place, and the resulting cell is called an 'induced pluripotent stem cell'. That is, a cell that has been induced by researchers into becoming a pluripotent stem cell, and which can now give rise to all other cells.

As we've discussed, *natural* pluripotent stem cells are found at the beginning of life. This means their biological age is pretty much zero. So, scientists wondered whether *induced* pluripotent stem cells were young as well, or if they were still the same age as the adult cells from which they were derived. Using the epigenetic clock, it is clear that the Yamanaka factors do, in fact, turn back biological age. When scientists use the Yamanaka factors in an adult cell, and the cell gradually transitions into an induced pluripotent stem cell, its biological age moves towards zero. Just like the age of a *natural* pluripotent stem cell. This is the closest we get to the backwards ageing of the jellyfish *Turritopsis* which is actually believed to happen with a similar mechanism.

Think about it for a second. The Yamanaka factors essentially turn back the biological clock. We could take a cell from your skin right now and use the Yamanaka factors to make it much younger than the rest of you. Again, cellular anti-ageing and immortality is a current reality.

But once more, the big question is to what degree we can transfer it to the whole organism. Using the four Yamanaka factors in all our cells is not a viable solution – that would make every cell climb all the way down our developmental

tree and end up at the 'ball of cells' state. There'd be no muscle cells, brain cells and so on, and the body would simply
disintegrate. Instead, scientists are trying to use the Yamanaka
factors in short pulses. The idea is that cells would then be
rejuvenated, but not so far that they end up as pluripotent cells.
This is called 'cellular reprogramming', and so far, it has shown
promising results in mice. For instance, the first scientists using
the technique found that it could increase the regenerative
ability of old mice. Since then, other scientists have used cellular reprogramming to restore youthful vision in old mice.
These scientists adjusted the normal protocol, though, in an
effort to decrease cancer risk. You see, cellular reprogramming
suffers from the same risk as the experiments with telomerase.
Only this time, the cancer is far more horrific. What happens
is that cells that are 'de-developed' too far end up as pluripotent cells. These can then start development anew, forming a
cancer called a teratoma in the process. This cancer mimics
the growth of a new organism, which gives it some terrifying
characteristics. The tumour consists of all kinds of tissue. It
will often grow strands of hair, and for some reason, teratomas
often end up having teeth growing inside them as well. High
risk, high reward, right?

Many scientists and companies are, in fact, ready to take
the bet on cellular reprogramming. It's not hard to see why. A
lot of the other therapies we've discussed involve decreasing
some kind of damage or improving the ability to repair. That
means they might be able to postpone ageing or increase
health a little. Cellular reprogramming, on the other hand,
suggests some form of programmed ageing *and* a way to control the programme. That means it promises the ability to
turn age back and forth at will. We don't know how this is

going to pan out yet, but even the possibility is like a million dollars lying on the sidewalk. And of course, if you ever see that, I'd suggest you run really fast to get there first. Not surprisingly, this sidewalk race already has many contestants. Several companies backed by billionaires and big-name scientists have launched within a couple of years in the pursuit of cellular reprogramming in humans. Of particular note is the Silicon Valley start-up Altos Labs, which is potentially the biggest shot at fighting ageing anyone has ever taken. Investors have put $3 billion into the company, though exactly who is behind the money is unknown. Several of the richest people in the world, among them Jeff Bezos, are rumoured to be involved. As a result, the employee roll at Altos Labs is hard to distinguish from the literature list in the back of this book. The company has hired many of the best researchers of ageing in the world, and is betting that given sufficient funds, they will be able to turn cellular reprogramming into an actual Fountain of Youth.

★ ★ ★

Cellular reprogramming is not the only way in which the Yamanaka factors and pluripotent stem cells are relevant to the fight against ageing. As we've discussed, pluripotent stem cells have the ability to become any cell type in the body. So what if we learned how cells normally turn into, say, heart muscle cells, and then coaxed the pluripotent stem cells in that direction? Then we could essentially make spare parts for the body. We could take our pluripotent stem cells and, with the right knowledge, turn them into any cell type we need. Getting a kidney replacement would no longer be dependent on the kindness of family members, friends or strangers: instead, a new one could be made *with your own cells*. And we could potentially create 'replacement' organs for old age instead of tirelessly trying to rejuvenate the ones we have.

While this stuff might sound like science fiction, the research has actually been going on for decades already. Scientists are trying to make any cell or tissue type you can think of – even brain cells. Like so much of biology, though, this stuff is really hard. The stem cells are difficult to make, they are time-consuming to take care of, and the signalling molecules used to coax their development are often extremely expensive. So progress has been slow. But it is there. In fact, the decades of work are now finally starting to come to fruition. It will be a while before we can make entire replacement organs consisting of complex structures with many different cell types. But there has been a lot of progress in making individual types of cells. For instance, scientists at Harvard have succeeded in making what are called beta cells. These are cells of the pancreas that produce the hormone insulin. In type 1 diabetes, the beta cells are attacked by the immune system, which ultimately kills them. This used to be deadly, but today we can make artificial insulin so that patients themselves can take over the job of the beta cells. Tracking blood sugar and injecting insulin is a big nuisance, though, and merely treats the symptoms; it's not a cure. But with the development of beta cells from pluripotent stem cells, the cure is near. In fact, the first patient has already had 'artificial' beta cells transplanted and been cured of his type 1 diabetes.

The beta cell effort, and others like it, did not actually use *induced* pluripotent stem cells, though. Instead, they used what is called embryonic stem cells. These cells are *not* from the patient themselves, but actual cells from the 'ball of cells' state – the embryo. Because they are not the person's own cells, they can cause problems with the immune system. If the immune system discovers foreign cells, it will attack and kill them. This can be dangerous – even deadly – to the patient. And of course, it also defeats the purpose a little. If the immune system kills the new cells, we won't have much use of them. However, fortunately, we have lots of experience with organ transplantation, so we know how to keep the immune system at bay. And scientists are also working to modify the stem cells so that the immune system won't recognise and attack them. This still leaves one final concern, though. The embryonic stem cells are often derived from leftover embryos created for artificial insemination. This means they are from a potential human who was not born which raises an ethical dilemma: is it okay to use these cells, which are, in essence, from another human? It's a similar discussion to that concerning the cells of Henrietta Lacks. Both types of cells have helped tremendously in the development of medical therapies, saving countless lives in the process. But as always, technological development forces us to make ethical trade-offs and reflect on our values.

Besides the pluripotent stem cells present during development, there are also stem cells in the adult body. The vast majority of these are not 'pluripotent', though, but 'multipotent'. This means they can create several cell types but not all. The adult stem cells are tasked with replacing the cells that are continuously lost, either to damage or due to normal cell turnover. For instance, the outermost layer of your gut is replaced every four days, skin cells are replaced every ten to thirty days and red blood cells live approximately 120 days. Not all cell types are replaced this often; for instance, only ten per cent of the cells in your bones are replaced each year, and some cells, like your brain cells, typically last your entire life. But the general rule is that your cells need to be replaced occasionally, and that makes adult stem cells important.

In fact, your stem cells determine your ability to regenerate at tissue level. Autophagy and similar recycling or repair processes help individual cells recover from damage. But on a tissue level, repair and maintenance is taken care of by stem cells. Like so many other repair mechanisms in the body, though, the ability of your stem cells deteriorates over time. As we age, stem cells become passive and worse at making new cells to replace lost ones. This phenomenon is usually called 'stem cell exhaustion'. The result is that we get worse at recovering from injury as we age, and eventually even normal maintenance cannot be upheld. For instance, the stem cells responsible for making new immune cells get worse over time, and that is one of the reasons old people have weaker immune systems. They also take longer to recover from injuries or surgeries, while having a higher risk of long-term complications, all because the ability to regenerate worsens as stem cells give up.

So while we envision replacing entire organs with new ones made from pluripotent stem cells, we could also replace adult stem cells to increase regenerative ability. Even though it sounds like a scammy procedure from Hollywood, you can imagine getting stem cell injections to fight ageing. This approach is especially developed for what is called mesenchymal stem cells. These are stem cells that make cells of bone, muscle, cartilage and fat. In one experiment, researchers isolated mesenchymal stem cells from young mice and injected them into old mice. Originally, the research was meant to examine if mesenchymal stem cell injections could be a treatment for osteoporosis, a disease of old age in which bones lose density and become weaker. One reason for this disease could be that stem cells don't produce the cells required for maintenance. To the researchers' surprise, though, their treatment didn't just affect bone health. It actually also made the mice live longer. While that doesn't necessarily mean it would help people in the same way, some plastic surgeons actually already use mesenchymal stem cells to regenerate sun-damaged skin, while there are clinics that offer treatments for various sports injuries with mesenchymal stem cells.

So, whether we're talking cellular reprogramming, organ replacements or stem cell injections, there is no doubt stem cell research will be delivering a lot of future therapies against ageing.

Chapter 13
Bloody Marvellous

In the early 1920s, a troubled Soviet scientist wandered around Moscow with big visions for the future of humanity.

Alexander Bogdanov, as he was called, was a writer, philosopher, physician, and committed communist – not just the kind who's afraid of ending up in Siberia, but someone who would make even the proudest comrades blush. Inspired by his own sci-fi novels, his political ideals and his studies of single-celled organisms, Bogdanov was convinced that humans ought to share blood with each other. This would be a necessary step towards the ideal communist society, and Bogdanov suspected it would double as a cure for ageing. Ever a man of action, he used his political sway in the Kremlin and was soon given the opportunity to found an institute for blood transfusions in Moscow. Bogdanov wasted no time and started conducting transfusions right away, of course using himself as one of the test subjects.

In the beginning, everything went according to plan. Bogdanov participated in ten blood transfusions over two years and considered them a success. One friend even remarked that he thought Bogdanov looked ten years younger than his actual age. Eventually, though, Bogdanov's luck ran out, and his eleventh blood transfusion went horribly wrong. To this day, we still don't know exactly what happened. The blood transfusion partner had both malaria and tuberculosis, Bogdanov had an immune reaction to the blood itself and all of this took place in a country where political figures made a virtue out of murdering each other in the most creative and imaginative ways possible.

Whatever happened, Bogdanov died two weeks after the blood transfusion at the age of fifty-four, following complications of the kidneys and the heart.

★ ★ ★

Alexander Bogdanov was far from the first scientist to experiment with blood transfusions. And in fact, his level of eccentricity wasn't that unusual in the field either. Blood transfusion experiments started all the way back in 1864, when French scientist Paul Bert thought it would be a good idea to sew two mice together – probably, at least in part, to show that he could. This unsavoury experiment paid off, in that Bert discovered how the circulatory systems of mice would automatically fuse after the operation, meaning the conjoined mice began to share blood. This peculiar phenomenon was dubbed parabiosis, and over the next few decades, other scientists occasionally ventured there as well. Among other things, their experiments helped clear the way for successful organ transplantations.

Despite the many eccentric people involved, though, it took almost 100 years from Bert's initial experiments before scientists researched the use of parabiosis to combat ageing. American researcher Clive McCay was among the first when he tried stitching together pairs of old and young mice to see how they would affect each other. These experiments never went far, though, and soon faded into obscurity. But then in 2005, the concept resurfaced in a research group at Stanford University. Once again, the scientists sewed together two mice of different ages. They found that the pairing increased the regenerative ability of the old mouse – rejuvenated it – while simultaneously weakening the young mouse. In other words, the two mice seemed to converge towards each other's physical states when sharing blood. Such a finding might make sense in a fantasy novel about vampires, but the scientists were quite puzzled. How could blood somehow transfer regenerative ability? Some believed youthful stem cells would travel from the young mouse and take up residence in the old mouse. Those young stem cells might then explain why the old mouse suddenly fared better. However, that turned out not to be the case. The regeneration actually comes from the old mouse's own stem cells. It seems young blood can somehow make old stem cells lighten up and start acting young again. The effect has nothing to do with blood cells either, as studies show all that is needed for rejuvenation is blood *plasma* – the blood minus its cells. The remaining fluid is full of all kinds of hormones and nutrients, as well as various proteins. We already know that the composition of blood plasma changes as we age, but many scientists used to believe this was just a downstream effect of ageing. The parabiosis experiments offer a clue that the arrow of causation might point the other way as well: maybe changes to blood plasma *contribute* to ageing rather than just track it.

★ ★ ★

The story of rejuvenation through young blood has not been lost on entrepreneurs. After all, it would be pretty easy to pay some young people to donate blood and then sell the blood at high margins to elderly millionaires. Blood transfusions are a common medical procedure, so it wouldn't be hard to find qualified staff either. A US company with this exact business plan, called Ambrosia (not the custard brand), opened its doors in 2016. But it was closed after the Food and Drug Administration issued a warning notice. We simply don't know enough about this stuff yet to declare any sort of medical benefits. Claims about 'immortality', didn't help the company's credibility, either.

Fortunately, other companies are using this research in more rigorous ways. These companies hope to identify which factors in young blood are responsible for the rejuvenating effect seen in old mice. We know it can't be the cells, so most likely it is some kind of soluble protein. If we're lucky, it's a single protein, or just a few. If we're unlucky, this is one of those impossible biological labyrinths where everything affects everything else. If that's the case, the solution might be to stick with blood plasma rather than trying to narrow it down any further. There are currently clinical trials investigating both of these approaches. A few have even concluded and published their results. For instance, there was one trial in which Alzheimer's patients received blood plasma from young people. Drumroll . . . it didn't work.

Research into young blood is still ongoing, but new studies cast doubt on what exactly explains the rejuvenating effect. It's certainly possible that young blood contains what we could call 'anti-ageing factors' – molecules that keep us young. But it turns out the constitution of *old* blood might be more important. You see, studies show it's not actually necessary to replace old blood with young blood to rejuvenate old mice. You can get the same effect by replacing the blood with a simple saline solution containing a little protein. That is, old mice are equally rejuvenated if you simply draw a little blood and replace the fluid with some protein-containing salt water. This suggests what really matters in these experiments is not what you add but what you *take away*. Old blood must contain 'pro-ageing factors' that burden the mice and that it is beneficial to remove.

This finding is especially interesting because we know of a natural experiment in humans with which we can compare it: blood donation. In a typical blood donation, you lose approximately half a litre of blood. Initially, your body will replace the lost blood volume with fluid from the rest of the body, and then during the following weeks, it will replenish the blood cells and various blood components. That means blood donors have a somewhat similar experience to the old mice in the saline experiments. If occasional removal of some blood has any kind of life-extending effect, we should be able to detect it in blood donors. A Danish study has looked for just this effect – and found it. It turns out blood donors actually live longer than other people. This effect persists even when you account for the fact that blood donors might be healthier at baseline. After all, they were well enough to be allowed to start donating blood. And interestingly, the effect gets stronger the more blood donations a blood donor makes. Admittedly, the effect is moderate – you're not going to live forever because you start donating blood. But given that it would be a good thing to do anyway, it's worth consideration.

> # Bloodletting is back
> The connection between bloodletting and health is not
> new. For much of history, bloodletting was a common
> medical practice but for some reason often performed by
> barbers. It used to be normal to visit your barber for a
> haircut and then subsequently have a little blood drawn.
> In fact, the red line in barbershop poles represents the
> blood that used to be drawn at barbershops. At the time,
> people prescribed all sorts of health benefits to regular
> bloodletting, but the belief was based on folk wisdom, not
> scientific research. As a result, bloodletting was used for
> *everything*. Even gunshot wounds.

So where could the health benefits of donating blood come
from? One possibility is good old hormesis. Losing half a litre
of blood is a stress factor to the body – and one it's easy to
imagine we've evolved to handle. Nowadays, losing blood is
rare, but people used to have all sorts of bloodsucking intestinal
parasites, as well as a tendency to fight each other with various
sharp objects. However, as we've discussed, it is also possible
that old blood contains 'pro-ageing factors' – certain molecules
that somehow promote ageing and that we benefit from getting rid of. If that's the case, there are thousands of possible
culprits. But one of the interesting ones is iron.

It works like this: when you donate blood, you lose a lot of
red blood cells. These are the cells you use to transport oxygen from the lungs around the body. Red blood cells transport oxygen using a specific protein called haemoglobin, and
inside every haemoglobin protein sit iron molecules. In fact, it
is iron that gives red blood cells – and by extension blood itself

– that red colour. Thus, when donating blood, you lose a lot of iron-containing red blood cells, which have to be replaced. As you're making the new red blood cells, you use iron from cellular deposits to make haemoglobin, and in that way blood donation lowers iron levels.

Now, losing a lot of iron might not sound particularly healthy. After all, we usually warn people about getting too *little* iron. But iron actually appears in some pretty ghastly circumstances. For instance, people with Alzheimer's and Parkinson's disease have abnormal amounts of iron in the diseased areas of the brain, and Alzheimer's progresses more rapidly in those with particularly high brain-iron levels. Similarly, there are abnormal amounts of iron in the plaque that accumulates in blood vessels with age, and which can cause heart attacks and strokes. There was even a randomised controlled trial where doctors decreased people's cancer risk by lowering their iron levels using blood draws. The trial had 1,300 participants who were divided into two groups. One periodically had blood drawn while the other did not. When the trial ended, cancer cases were thirty-five per cent lower among those who had regularly had blood drawn. And those in the blood-drawing group who did get cancer had a sixty per cent increased chance of surviving.

Genetic studies also back up the association between iron metabolism and longevity. Do you remember Genome-Wide Association Studies (GWAS) from earlier? These are studies where scientists identify what genetic variants cause our different traits. We learned that genetic variants affecting the immune system, growth, metabolism and the generation of zombie cells were implicated in ageing. But besides that, these studies actually also implicate iron. At least, people genetically prone to higher iron levels seem to die earlier than others. This finding is backed up by actual blood measurements. In a study on 9,000 Danes, scientists looked at a protein called ferritin, which is responsible for storing iron in our bodies. The more iron you have in your body, the higher your ferritin levels will be. And in the Danish study, researchers found that high ferritin levels were associated with a greater risk of an early death – especially among men.

Now, all this doesn't mean that *low* iron levels aren't dangerous, too. They very much are, especially for premenopausal women who lose a little blood – and thereby iron – every month. But the danger of excess iron exposes a flaw in how we often think about health. *More is better*. People take all kinds of supplements, because why not get a little extra of everything? That's the reasoning behind taking multivitamins, too. Maybe we're deficient, so better get some more of *everything*. Unfortunately, biology just doesn't work like that. A good example of the faults in this approach is laid out in a large study called the Iowa Women's Health Study. Here, scientists followed 39,000 women and found, among other things, that those taking iron supplements had a higher risk of dying early than those who didn't. The same was true for those taking a multivitamin pill, which of course contains iron.

To be fair, the reason the 'more is better' approach doesn't cause problems more often is that our bodies do a pretty good job of regulating most nutrients and vitamins. In many cases, your body can excrete something if you get too much. But iron is one of the exceptions. Your body actually has no system for excreting excess iron. You passively lose a little through sweat, dead cells and bleeding, but there is no dedicated mechanism for pumping out iron if you suddenly have too much. The reason is probably that iron excess never used to be a problem in the past, because of lower dietary intakes, blood-sucking intestinal parasites and more frequent bleeding. Today, though, it's another story, and men especially can be prone to accumulate iron with age. An extreme example is the genetic disease hereditary haemochromatosis. This genetic disease makes the affected absorb more iron than usual from their food. If not diagnosed and treated, people with haemochromatosis eventually end up with sky-high iron levels. As a result, they usually die early from cancer or heart complications, and before that start suffering from all kinds of maladies, such as diabetes, fatigue and joint pain. Unless, that is, if they have their iron levels lowered using blood draws, in which case the condition is harmless.

The Celtic curse or the Viking disease?

Hereditary haemochromatosis (HH) is almost exclusively found in Europeans. It was once nicknamed 'the Celtic Curse' because there's a particularly high frequency of the disease in Ireland. Another theory is that the disease was spread by the Vikings. There's a high frequency of HH in Scandinavia, too, and scientists have noted disease frequency tends to be high in areas raided and settled by the Vikings. Like many other genetic diseases, the development of HH requires that you inherit a mutated version of the implicated gene from both parents. If you inherit only one HH genetic variant, you'll be fine. HH is obviously not evolutionarily advantageous, but scientists suspect the genetic variant might have become common anyway because there can be benefits to carrying a single copy. That is, perhaps the HH genetic variant persisted because those with a single copy fared better than the average person, even though those with two copies fared worse. The benefit in question could be helping farmers survive on grain-heavy diets that are low in iron. But there are other possibilities, too. The mechanism could be that slightly higher iron levels lead to a higher volume of red blood cells and thus a higher aerobic ability.

For instance, one study found that eighty per cent of medal-winning French athletes at world-class competitions have a single version of the HH genetic variant even though a lot fewer normal French people have it. And other studies have shown that being a carrier of one copy of the HH genetic variant is associated with improved physical endurance compared to non-carriers.

There must be a reason why excess iron shows up in all the wrong places. One possibility is that iron promotes the formation of free radicals. It is well known that iron stimulates our metaphorical bull in a china shop. Yes, we've learned that free radicals are not as big an issue as scientists once thought. In low doses, they're even beneficial, as they work through hormesis. However, as always, hormesis is about the dose. If you exceed the level of damage that the body can repair, a stressor becomes net damaging and lowers lifespan.

But there's another possibility that can explain the iron-longevity connection, too: microorganisms *love* iron. Iron is necessary for all living creatures, and microbes such as bacteria and fungi are no exception. In fact, iron works almost like fertiliser for the growth of bacteria. The difference between a harmless and a life-threatening infection can be how good the bacteria is at procuring iron for itself – or how much iron is available. This has caused troubles in underdeveloped countries, where many children are iron-deficient. Growing up with iron deficiency can stunt growth and cognitive development, so the World Health Organization recommends iron supplements to combat the deficiency. However, iron supplements can come with the downside of increasing children's risk of getting malaria and various bacterial infections – and the supplements can also increase the severity of disease once infected.

Evolution has actually already built this knowledge into our bodies. Access to iron is one of the most important battlefields when fighting infections. If your immune system detects an infection, the body immediately turns up the production of the iron-storage protein ferritin. That way, iron can be locked away in what is essentially a molecular cage so that microbes can't get to it. Similarly, infections also make your body increase the production of a protein called hepcidin, which blocks iron uptake from your food. So perhaps it's time we take a closer look at the world of microbes.

Chapter 14
Microbe Struggles

In 1847, the Hungarian-German physician Ignaz Semmelweis was trudging around Vienna with a burdened conscience.

Semmelweis was an obstetrician, a doctor specialising in pregnancy and childbirth, and was in charge of the maternity ward at Vienna General Hospital. The hospital had set up two clinics to offer free maternity care to the poor women of the city. And in return, one of the clinics was used to train new midwives while the other was used to train new doctors.

To Semmelweis's dismay, there was a large difference in maternal mortality rates between the two clinics. At the midwife-training facility, four per cent of mothers died during childbirth, but at the facility training new doctors, more than ten per cent of mothers perished. The cause was a mysterious disease called 'childbed fever'.

The poor women of Vienna were well aware of the different mortality rates. They begged and pleaded to be taken to the safer clinic when going into labour. Some even chose to give birth on the street rather than risk ending up in the hands of the young doctors.

Semmelweis was deeply unhappy about the situation, and did everything in his power to identify the cause. He tried to align all procedures and instruments between the two clinics, but mortality rates just didn't budge.

One day, Semmelweis's friend Jakob Kolletschka was accidentally cut by a student's scalpel while he was performing an autopsy. The cut gave Kolletschka a bad infection, and not long afterwards, he passed away. At his autopsy, doctors found suspicious similarities to the women with 'childbed fever' and then, something finally clicked for Ignaz Semmelweis.

Back then, it was normal for doctors to go straight from conducting autopsies to attending deliveries: that is, from cutting open dead people to assisting women in childbirth. Semmelweis became convinced there was a connection; he reasoned doctors transferred 'cadaverous particles' from corpses to the expecting mothers. After some reflection, he suggested that the particles could be removed by handwashing with calcium hypochlorite (the 'chlorine' used today for disinfecting swimming pools). He immediately made it obligatory for all doctors at the hospital to wash their hands before getting anywhere near the women in childbirth.

The new initiative provided the breakthrough Semmelweis had sought, and the mortality rate at the hospital plummeted. In April, just before the introduction of handwashing, 18.7 per cent of expecting mothers passed away. By June, only 2.2 per cent did. And by July, mortality rates had dropped all the way down to 1.2 per cent.

Semmelweis immediately set about reporting his discovery to the medical community. This was a big deal and could save countless lives. However, to Semmelweis's surprise, the reception was mostly hostile. Some doctors were deeply offended that he would even suggest they were unclean. Others pointed out that Semmelweis's observations didn't fit the prominent scientific theories of the day.

One critic was the respected Danish obstetrician Carl Levy, who also struggled with sky-high maternal mortality rates in Copenhagen. Levy wrote that it was absurd to think that something microscopically small – so small you couldn't even *see* it – could cause such a serious disease. The numbers from Vienna had to be a coincidence.

For years, poor Semmelweis fought the criticism hailing down on him from all directions. He wrote letter after letter to prominent people in the medical establishment but to no avail. The resistance eventually made him so furious that he accused his opponents of being murderers. Before long, he turned any conversation towards maternal mortality and handwashing.

As time went on, Semmelweis's mental state began deteriorating. In 1861, he developed severe depression, and soon after began to experience nervous breakdowns. A few years later, he was admitted to a psychiatric institution. Here, he was beaten by the guards, developed an infection, and – ironically – died of blood poisoning at the age of forty-seven.

★ ★ ★

Around the time of Semmelweis's death, there were, fortunately, other people making strides in microbiology too. A trifecta of scientists from the European 'big three' – France, Britain and Germany – helped to establish the theory that microbes can cause disease. First, the Frenchman Louis Pasteur proved that microbes don't arise out of thin air, as was commonly believed at the time. He also discovered that microbes are the cause of fermentation in beer and wine (the process that makes alcohol), and that microbes make food rot.

Food decay can be avoided in three different ways, Pasteur demonstrated: by using high heat (pasteurisation), by filtration, or by applying chemical solutions. This gave the English surgeon Joseph Lister an idea. Back then, patients often got infections after surgeries. Lister thought that chemical solutions might be used to avoid this, and developed methods to sterilise surgical equipment and wounds. Subsequently, the German scientist Robert Koch developed methods for growing bacteria in the laboratory, and finally started linking specific bacteria to the development of particular diseases, such as tuberculosis, cholera and anthrax.

Of course, all this progress happened under constant critical assault – but, over time, the evidence became irrefutable. Even the most stubborn critics had to yield.

It might be hard for us today to understand how people used to believe bacteria arose out of thin air, or how doctors thought it was fine to commute between corpses and patients without washing their hands. But the steep opposition to new ideas hits closer to home.

Today, we've developed an arsenal of weapons against microbes. We have antibiotics that can kill almost all the bacteria that used to haunt us. We have vaccines that can protect us from diseases that used to be deadly or incapacitating. And we have tons of knowledge of hygiene, paths of infection and sterility.

At one point, it even seemed like we could declare the final victory in our ancient battle against microbes.

But is that true?

★ ★ ★

In the early 1980s in Perth, Australia, a pathologist named Robin Warren noticed something strange in laboratory samples from peptic ulcer patients. When examining them closely, he could see small, spiral-shaped bacteria in all of them. Warren approached a young doctor named Barry Marshall, who immediately began investigating.

At the time, people *knew* that peptic ulcers were caused by stress. They definitely didn't have anything to do with bacteria. Most scientists assumed that the spiral-shaped bacteria Robin Warren found must have originated in the laboratory. There had probably been contamination of the samples. However, Warren and Marshall weren't convinced, and decided to continue studying the mysterious microbes.

The first step was to isolate the bacteria and grow them in the laboratory. The two scientists gathered 100 patients with peptic ulcers and took biopsies from all of them. The effort was a disappointment, though, as no bacterial colonies grew from the samples. This continued in successive tries until luck finally shone on the Australians. Normally, patient samples were allowed to grow on Petri dishes for two days, as was the custom at the time. But on one occasion, one of the Petri dishes was left for a full six days because the scientists had their Easter holiday. That was enough time for a colony of spiral-shaped bacteria to develop.

Warren and Marshall were convinced that they'd found the real cause of peptic ulcers. It wasn't stress, diet, lack of exercise, nor anything else that the textbooks claimed. Instead, it was all down to these small, spiral-shaped bacteria.

The two Australians shared their discovery with anyone who would listen, but the reception was mostly cold. Their peers argued that bacterial diseases were a thing of the past; they'd all been identified decades ago and cured with the invention of antibiotics. Now, scientists were working with much more sophisticated theories. It was no longer cool to look for bacteria – and by the way, it couldn't possibly be as simple as the two Australians claimed. Bacteria would never even be able to survive the harsh gastric acid.

Besides, everyone already *knew* what caused peptic ulcers, and there was a large industry specialising in alleviating the symptoms using antacids. At the time, two to four per cent of Americans had antacids in their pockets, so this was *big business*.

★ ★ ★

As it turns out, Warren and Marshall weren't the first scientists to posit a link between infection and peptic ulcers. In the late 1800s, several researchers observed bacteria in laboratory samples from peptic ulcer patients. And at the dawn of the next century, Japanese researchers even brought on peptic ulcers in guinea pigs by using some suspicious spiral-shaped bacteria they had isolated from cats.

The theory never took hold, though, and the last bit of hope was extinguished in the 1950s when a famous pathologist decided to test it. He searched for bacteria in peptic ulcer patients, but found none because he'd used the wrong method.

Afterwards, the idea slipped out of the scientific consciousness, although it occasionally re-emerged – for instance, when a Greek doctor treated his own peptic ulcer with antibiotics and successfully used the method on his patients as well. No scientific journals wanted to publish his findings, though, and no drug companies were interested in the treatment. As a thanks, the Greek authorities fined the doctor and took him to court.

So, opposition to the bacterial theory of peptic ulcers was nothing new. Warren and Marshall managed to convince a couple of microbiologists who thought bacteria were the most fascinating thing ever. But other than that, their theory got drowned out by publication after publication with claims about stress, diet, gastric acid and so on.

It didn't help that the two Australians had trouble demonstrating their theory in animals. When they tried to infect anything from pigs to mice, the spiral-shaped bacteria simply refused to take hold.

In time, Warren and Marshall grew desperate. They knew they were on to something, and could even cure their patients with antibiotics. So could the rest of the world's doctors, but only if Warren and Marshall managed to convince the necessary authorities. The only option was to prove their theory in humans once and for all. But how?

With pure Australian nerve, Barry Marshall decided to use himself as a guinea pig. He isolated the spiral-shaped bacteria from a patient, let them grow established in a culture – and then swallowed them. After a few days, he became well and truly ill. Ten days later, the bacteria had spread throughout his stomach, giving him a precursor to peptic ulcers. And, after careful documentation, Marshall used antibiotics to eradicate the infection and cure himself.

The daring self-experiment was enough to finally turn the tide in the Australians' favour. It would be another ten years before the last resistance was swept off the field (and the patent on antacids expired). However, the spiral bacterium, *Helicobacter pylori*, was gradually recognised as the primary cause of peptic ulcers, and also as the cause of most cases of stomach cancer.

Victory was sweet for the stubborn Australians. In 2005, Robin Warren and Barry Marshall were awarded the greatest honour in science, the Nobel Prize, for their discovery.

Once upon a time, our understanding of how microbes cause disease went something like this: you get infected with a specific microbe, for instance a bacterium or a virus, and then you develop a corresponding disease. This was one of the reasons Robin Warren and Barry Marshall met resistance. They were working to prove that the bacterium *Helicobacter pylori* causes peptic ulcers and stomach cancer. But some people carry *Helicobacter pylori* in their stomachs with no problems. Nevertheless, the bacterium *is* the cause, and its eradication is a treatment. It simply turns out that the relationship between us and microbes is a lot more complicated than we once thought.

Back in the day, we used to think humans were mostly sterile. But in recent decades, technological advancement has revealed that's anything but true. We're actually teeming with trillions of non-human organisms – what is called the 'microbiome'. In fact, there are more cells of foreign origin in your body than there are your own. These organisms (counting bacteria, viruses, fungi and others) live on your skin, in your mouth, in your intestinal system and everywhere in between. You can imagine the situation as something similar to a tree in the rainforest. While the tree may have preferred to be left alone, it is home to all sorts of insects, reptiles, birds, mammals and even other plants. In the same way, you're not just a person, but an entire ecosystem of living things.

Among your microbial guests are those that are beneficial to you. There are also those that don't affect you all that much. And finally, there are those you'd rather be without. The beneficial microbes include bacteria that perform important biological functions, for instance, bacteria in the intestinal system that aid your digestion. One example is bacteria that use indigestible dietary fibre to make a health-promoting compound called butyrate. Another example is the bacteria we've previously met that produce the autophagy-promoting compound spermidine. But there are also other – much weirder – examples of microbes helping us out, such as gut bacteria that can help runners improve their endurance by breaking down lactate so that it doesn't build up.

There are also microbes that are primarily helpful because they protect us against *other* microbes. You see, the ecosystem in your gut (and elsewhere) is balanced by competition for food and space. Gut bacteria will actively try to crowd each other out, fight each other and even eat each other. Some disorders of the gut arise when this balance gets disrupted, for instance, when a course of antibiotics kill beneficial bacteria, allowing harmful ones to vastly expand their real estate.

While it might sound nice and cosy to think that some microbes are helping you, I want to stress that this is not due to some kind of empathy. The microbes in your body are interested in themselves and themselves only. As you are their home, it can sometimes be beneficial for them to help you out. But if conditions change, and they can get a leg-up at your expense, they'll gladly do so.

For example, imagine a harmless bacterium coexisting peacefully somewhere in your body. The bacterium reproduces occasionally but is also kept in check by your immune system. At one point, a mutation changes the bacterium, allowing it to suddenly evade your immune system. This will probably allow the bacterium to make many more copies of itself and could help it beat its competitors and more easily spread to new hosts. This will come at your expense, though, as the bacterium starts using up valuable resources and may even hurt you in the process. Obviously, if the bacterium goes so far that it ends up killing you, it will lose its home. But even that can sometimes be an acceptable price in evolutionary terms, if it helps the bacterium spread. It's a devilish and egoistic strategy, but of course not due to actual sentience. It's just simple evolution. Microbes that manage to produce more copies of themselves prevail.

The most popular place for microbes to settle is on the skin and in the gastrointestinal tract. Here they have access to food, and there is less immune activity because both are a surface of the body rather than its inside (there's a hole from the mouth and all the way through, so these surfaces are technically 'outside' too). But it is not only on the 'outer' surfaces of the body that microbes take up residence. In fact, it turns out that even the organs we once thought were sterile abound with life.

Take blood, for example. Until recently, medical science assumed that our blood was sterile. But we now know that's not true. When you incubate blood samples from blood donors under the right conditions, you can grow all sorts of different microbes from it. (Maybe the secret of young blood is that it has fewer harmful microbes?)

The brain is an even more extreme example. Previously, it was thought that the brain had to be sterile because it is protected by something called the blood–brain barrier. As the name suggests, the blood–brain barrier is a barrier that separates the blood from the brain. Oxygen and nutrients can pass through, but it's notoriously difficult for most molecules to enter the brain. This is one of the reasons why it is so difficult to develop drugs for mental illnesses. The brain is our most important organ, so it makes sense that we want to protect it and keep microbes out.

That said, there *are* microbes in the brain. Actually, scientists have identified more than 200 different kinds already – and they're not done looking. Really, there are microbes in any place you can imagine – and we could continue with microbes in the muscles, in the liver, in the chest and so on.

The point is that all these microbes don't just sit around. They affect everything that happens in your body. In fact, they even affect our medical efforts. Studies show that at least half of the most popular drugs are altered by bacteria before they even enter the body from the gut.

The life-extending, brain-controlling parasite

There's a certain kind of parasite – a tapeworm – that cycles between birds and ants. The tapeworm lives in the guts of birds like woodpeckers, and its eggs are excreted in the birds' faeces. When ants eat the contaminated faeces, the parasites hatch and take up residence in the ant's abdomen. Here, they have a steady stream of nutrients on which to live. However, the parasites ultimately aim to return to the gut of a bird, as this is the only place where they can lay eggs. It's a weird lifecycle. To achieve their goal, the tapeworms completely take control of the ant. The positive side – if there's ever such a thing when infected with brain-controlling parasites – is that the tapeworms have found a way to prolong the lives of their hosts. Parasitised ants live at least three times longer than non-infected ants.

We don't really know how it all works, though. And of course, the parasites are not trying to be helpful. They just want the ant to live longer, so it has a higher chance of being eaten by a bird at some point. And if a bird does show up, the parasites leave their host no mercy. The tapeworm thwarts the ant's natural fear response so instead of fleeing, the parasitised ant just sits around helplessly while staring blankly at the sky.

Chapter 15
Hiding in Plain Sight

When the United States began vaccinating against the measles virus in the 1960s, children fortunately stopped getting measles. But that wasn't the only thing; suddenly, American children had plummeting risks of dying from all sorts of other infectious diseases, too. The same thing happened in European countries joining the effort. But how can a vaccine protect against infections that it's not even targeting?

Like all other microbes that infect us, the measles virus is not a big fan of our immune system. Cells of the immune system are constantly on the lookout for invaders and will spring into action if an uninvited guest is discovered. Viruses like the measles virus fight back by hiding, by trying to trick the immune system and sometimes also by counterattack. This war between our immune system and various microbes is ongoing throughout our lives. It's happening inside you at this very moment.

Pathogens have evolved various weapons to target the immune system, but the measles virus has found a particularly effective one. It can cause something you can think of as immune memory loss. Usually, certain cells of the immune system retain a memory of previous adversaries. This is clever, because it decreases the time it takes for the immune system to react if it encounters the same enemy again. Then, there will already be a tried-and-tested battleplan ready for deployment to rob the infection of the chance to take hold. This immune 'memory' is the reason vaccines can protect against developing a disease, and also the reason you only get diseases such as chickenpox once in a lifetime.

When the measles virus causes 'memory loss' in our immune system, though, all this valuable information is lost. This benefits the measles virus itself, but it's also a boon for all sorts of other bacteria and viruses. Suddenly, these pathogens have a much easier time infecting us. Therefore, infection with the measles virus predisposes you to all sorts of other infections, too. In fact, it is estimated that the measles virus used to contribute to half of childhood deaths from *other* infections.

Such one-two punches are quite common in the world of infections. A straight right from an initial infection and then a left hook from a second one that exploits the chaos to its own benefit. On the one hand, this principle illustrates why vaccines were (and still are) the uncrowned king of medical science. But it is also bad news, because there are still plenty of dangerous microbes that we don't have vaccines against yet.

A particularly good example is HIV, the virus that causes AIDS. HIV attacks certain cells of the immune system called T-cells. You can think of T-cells as the generals of the immune system, because they are responsible for orchestrating your immune responses. When HIV attacks T-cells, they eventually succumb to the virus. This means the immune system becomes weaker and weaker, and eventually it cannot keep up with all sorts of other microbes. As a result, HIV-infected people become vulnerable to otherwise harmless infections. Microbes, which normally live in or on us in peaceful coexistence, sense an opportunity and begin to grow out of control. The relatively harmless fungus *Candida albicans* – which lives on over half of us – can turn into a serious infection. Herpes virus 8 can go from being relatively harmless to causing a form of cancer called Kaposi's sarcoma. Even the flu can become deadly.

The infectious burden of HIV is taxing on the body, and even though we now have anti-HIV drugs that help patients live much longer than previously, they still die earlier than non-infected people. They also have an increased risk of everything from cancer to cardiovascular diseases. And in fact, it turns out that HIV infection in itself increases the rate of biological ageing. Patients with HIV are five to seven years older biologically than their actual age as measured by the epigenetic clock.

★ ★ ★

Fortunately, we're still making progress in the fight against HIV, and it is less of a health threat than it used to be. If you take normal precautions, getting infected is highly unlikely. However, there are other much more common infections that can similarly accelerate ageing. In fact, it looks like being infected in and of itself makes us grow old faster. The more and the worse infections you have, the quicker you age. This is probably one of the reasons why people today look so much younger than similarly aged people in the past. A hundred years ago, middle-aged people had lived a life ravished by infections from childhood. That means they looked older – and, frankly, more worn out – than middle-aged people today who have lived a life protected by vaccines.

While we've used vaccines to eradicate many of the viruses that used to kill and maim us, there are still nasty ones around today. One example is a virus called *cytomegalovirus* (CMV).

You've probably never heard of it before, but it's actually a very common viral infection. In developing countries, virtually everyone is infected by the time they reach adulthood. In the developed world, infection rates are lower, but the majority of people are still infected at some point in their life.

CMV is a member of the herpes virus family, along with the viruses that cause cold sores. You won't get cold sores from CMV, but like other herpes viruses, it's chronic. Once infected, you can never get rid of it again.

CMV is transmitted person-to-person through body fluids and can infect many different cell types in our bodies. After forcing access to a cell, the virus integrates into the cell's DNA and hijacks the cell for its own purposes. Then it enters a lifecycle that alternates between activity and dormancy. When active, CMV forces infected cells to produce more CMV particles, which can be used to spread the infection to new cells or to new individuals. Our immune system notices when CMV is causing trouble and will try to fight back. However, at any point CMV can retreat back into dormancy, which helps it escape. Then it will hide and wait for its next opportunity to awaken. The chronic nature of a CMV infection drives the immune system absolutely nuts. In infected individuals, up to ten per cent of key immune cells can be occupied trying to contain the virus. That obviously depletes the resources of the immune system and distracts it from other enemies. In this way, CMV increases the likelihood of many other infections.

You're unlikely to notice any of this, as CMV infections are mostly asymptomatic (except in babies, where they are the leading cause of hearing loss). However, using epigenetic clocks, scientists have found that a CMV infection accelerates the ageing process. It also seems to increase blood pressure long-term and might even promote the development of plaque in arteries. In addition, CMV prevents infected cells from carrying out cellular suicide, increasing their risk of becoming harmful zombie cells.

All of this makes CMV an obvious candidate for eradication by vaccination. However, just as it dodges our actual immune systems, it has also managed to dodge our 'extended' immune systems – medical science and the pharmaceutical industry. CMV is annoyingly hard to target, and as it has health consequences that are hidden at first glance, it wasn't taken seriously enough in the past. Now, though, vaccine efforts have picked up.

Another example of a pathogen that can accelerate the ageing process and lead to disease is CMV's cousin from the herpes virus family, Epstein-Barr virus (EBV). EBV is also chronic, and it is the virus that causes mononucleosis. It infects pretty much everyone before they reach adulthood. Those who don't get mononucleosis were typically infected with EBV in childhood, when symptoms are less severe and similar to those of a cold.

When infecting us, EBV especially targets cells of the immune system called B-cells. In rare cases, the virus makes these cells become cancerous as it takes control of them. However, that's not the only harm done by EBV. The virus has long been suspected of causing a whole range of autoimmune diseases, including multiple sclerosis, lupus, type 1 diabetes, rheumatoid arthritis and several others. A large-scale study of American military personnel has provided powerful proof that at the very least, the connection of EBV to multiple sclerosis is valid. In the study, scientists found that EBV infection incurs a thirty-two-fold increased risk of developing the disease. As mentioned, this has been our suspicion for a long time, but it has been difficult to prove causation. First, because many people are infected with EBV *without* getting multiple sclerosis. And second, because there can be years between the initial infection and its consequences. Even fifteen years after being infected with EBV, it seems the risk of getting multiple sclerosis is still higher than normal for example.

Autoimmune diseases like multiple sclerosis are diseases where the immune system mistakenly targets the body. It might sound odd that an infection can make us do this to ourselves, but the reason is as fascinating as something horrible can be. As we've discussed, microbes really don't like the immune system and try to avoid it. Just as in the jungle, the best way to hide is camouflage. Bacteria and viruses can do this by evolving proteins that look a lot like our own. Your immune system is trained to recognise what your own cells and proteins look like so that it only attacks outsiders. This means pathogens can sometimes successfully hide by pretending to be a normal part of your body. However, if such a pathogen *is* recognised by your immune system, big trouble might ensue. Then, your immune system can mistakenly begin to attack your own cells because it has now learned that's what the enemy looks like. In this case and many others, the pathogen doesn't target us directly – but it doesn't care about us either, and so can end up causing a lot of damage in trying to reach its own goals.

Unfortunately, even though we now know a lot about the damage caused by common infections such as CMV and EBV, it is not easy to avoid either. Besides, it's quite likely you're already infected. However, it's still worthwhile exercising a little caution. For instance, CMV can infect people multiple times, and due to the chronic nature of the infection, each time just makes matters worse. Besides, CMV and EBV are probably just the tip of the iceberg. Consider, for instance, that the rate of premature babies plummeted around the world during the early corona-virus lockdowns. This was a notoriously hard time for various pathogens, as we made it a lot more difficult for infections to spread. So maybe the reason for the lack of premature babies is that premature birth has an as-yet unidentified viral cause or contributor. Or consider the coronavirus itself, which seems to increase the risk of developing everything from diabetes to various heart conditions.

As a whole, there are countless viruses that target humans, including ones we don't know about yet. It's not hard to imagine that some of these contribute to ageing or disease; nor is it difficult to envision that diseases, for which we haven't yet identified the cause, could turn out to have bacterial or viral involvement. Okay, it might not be particularly wise to become a paranoid hypochondriac either, but it's certainly worthwhile using a little common sense and of course, getting vaccinated.

Chapter 16

Flossing for Longevity

Alzheimer's disease is one of the worst fates that can befall an old person. The neurodegenerative disease slowly erases a lifetime of memories until patients cannot even remember the people they love. It's a devastating way to end a long life.

The disease is characterised by the appearance of protein plaques in the brain. These plaques consist of a peptide called amyloid beta, and you can think of them as little clumps. We don't know why the amyloid beta clumps form, but we do know they can lead to inflammation in the brain and that they eventually kill brain cells.

This gives us an obvious solution: remove the clumps, or even better, prevent them from occurring in the first place. That's easier said than done, of course, because the brain is protected by the blood–brain barrier. As we've discussed, this makes it notoriously hard to develop drugs for the brain. A drug doesn't just have to work – say be able to remove the amyloid beta clumps – it also has to be able to actually get into the brain. And that can only be achieved by scaling what's essentially a biological version of the Berlin Wall.

Despite all the difficulties, pharmaceutical companies *have* in fact succeeded in developing drugs that can prevent amyloid beta clumps from forming in the brain. They have even developed drugs that can *remove* them. But unfortunately, it doesn't help. Nothing does, really. The fight against Alzheimer's has cost billions of dollars, and thousands of our most talented scientists have dedicated their lives to it. Hundreds of potential drugs have been tested in clinical trials, but despite the gargantuan effort, we have nothing to show for it. Every single promising drug has failed. There's no cure – not even a little hope for spontaneous remission. The best we can do is to slightly delay the inevitable.

What could we possibly be missing? There must be something fundamental about Alzheimer's that we don't yet understand. How else can *everything* fail? It doesn't help our efforts that Alzheimer's disease – unlike virtually all other diseases – is unique to humans. Mice, for example, often get cancer, but they simply don't get Alzheimer's. In order to research Alzheimer's, scientists have had to artificially design mice reminiscent of human Alzheimer's patients. And then try to cure these mice in the hopes that the lessons can be transferred back to humans.

Are we perhaps wrong about the involvement of amyloid beta clumps in Alzheimer's? That's very unlikely. You see, we know that people with Down's syndrome have a much higher risk of getting Alzheimer's disease. They also tend to get it very early. Down's syndrome is caused by having an extra copy of chromosome 21, and on that chromosome sits the amyloid beta gene. This suggests that an increased amount of amyloid beta coincides with Alzheimer's. Scientists believe other people with Alzheimer's experience something similar. Either they produce more amyloid beta than normal, or perhaps they are worse at clearing it up. In both cases, amyloid beta is seen as a sort of waste product. We don't really know what its intended function is – we only know it from Alzheimer's disease. So essentially, the story goes: we have a protein with no purpose, and in old age, it makes clumps in the brain and kills us.

That's a little hard to believe. Especially because we're far from the only animal that has the amyloid beta protein. In fact, it's extremely well-preserved throughout the course of evolution. Monkeys have it, mice have it – even fish have it. And all of these animals have versions of the protein that are nearly identical to our own. That's usually a clue that a protein has an important function. If an animal is born with a mutation in an important gene, they tend to fare worse than others, meaning they will not contribute as much to the next generation. This means proteins tend to change only slowly if they are important and will often be similar across species.

So, if amyloid beta is important, what is its function? Most likely, it is to be a weapon against microbes. You see, scientists have discovered that amyloid beta kills microbes if you add it to microbial cultures in the laboratory. It does so by clumping around the microbe to neutralise and kill it while subsequently keeping it under lock just in case. It's a fascinating mechanism and not just something that happens in laboratory cultures. If scientists inject bacteria into the brains of mice, amyloid beta springs into action and forms clumps around the bacteria. As a result, mice lacking amyloid beta are killed by these bacterial injections, while mice that can use amyloid beta tend to survive. At the same time, we know from the genetics of Alzheimer's that the immune system plays some kind of role in disease development.

So we certainly have a smoking gun suggesting that Alzheimer's could have microbial involvement. Now all we need to know is who pulled the trigger.

A study from Taiwan provides the main suspect. The Taiwanese researchers discovered that people infected with the herpes virus are two-and-a-half times more likely to get Alzheimer's than those who aren't – that is, unless they are taking anti-herpes medication. This medication suppresses the virus, and interestingly, it also brings the risk of Alzheimer's back to normal. The case strengthens as several research groups have found traces of the herpes virus in brain tissue samples from deceased Alzheimer's patients (while being absent from controls). In one study, the virus was even found *inside* the amyloid beta clumps in Alzheimer's brains. Researchers can also duplicate the effect in the laboratory. If brain cells in culture are infected with herpes virus, amyloid beta clumps appear – unless anti-herpes medicine is also added. The connection could also explain a puzzling finding about the grandfather of the Alzheimer's risk genes. We have previously encountered the APOE gene in which a specific genetic variant increases the risk of Alzheimer's disease. It turns out the same genetic variant increases the risk of getting cold sores for people infected with the herpes virus. It could be that this particular genetic variant simply makes people worse at fighting herpes infections.

Critics of the microbial theory of Alzheimer's point to the fact that some people are infected with herpes virus but *don't* develop Alzheimer's. But, as we've learned, this is quite normal. Some people are infected with *Helicobacter pylori* and don't get peptic ulcers. Some people are infected with Epstein-Barr virus and don't develop multiple sclerosis. In both cases, the disease happens as a by-product of infection – the pathogen is not trying to directly induce it. That's probably the reason why pathogens can cause disease in some people while sparing others. That, and the influence of genetics, different sub-strains, severity of infection and also randomness or luck.

The next critique point is more valid, though. As it turns out, the herpes virus is not the only pathogen that has been associated with the development of Alzheimer's disease. Suspect number two is the bacterium *Porphyromonas gingivalis* (*P. gingivalis*), which normally lives in the mouth. Again, *P. gingivalis* has been found in brain tissue from deceased Alzheimer's patients. In some cases, the bacterium can cause a severe inflammatory condition of the mouth called periodontitis. This condition is associated with an increased risk of Alzheimer's (and also of cardiovascular disease). In fact, there is even one study that gave dental examinations to 8,000 people in their sixties and found those with gum disease had a greater risk of developing dementia two decades down the line. Whether or not there is causation here, remember to floss.

Further down the list of suspects are the bacterium *Chlamydophila pneumoniae* (not to be confused with the sexually transmitted infection) and fungi such as *Candida albicans*. Again, both have been discovered in the brains of deceased Alzheimer's patients but not in controls. At this point, the best evidence is for the herpes virus, but as we've discussed already, one-two combinations from microbes are not uncommon. The culprit could be a single microbe with the rest being simple followers, it could be a combination, or microbes could turn out not to be the culprit after all. We don't yet know, but given that Alzheimer's is currently untreatable, it won't hurt to take the microbial theory seriously.

Infections messing up the brain

We already know other cases where infections cause Alzheimer's-like symptoms. One of these is syphilis, also known as the French, Italian or Spanish disease, depending on whether you ask the Italians, the French or the Portuguese. Syphilis is caused by a sexually transmitted bacterium that originated in the Americas but spread to the rest of the world after European contact. The bacterium found itself right at home, and before the invention of antibiotics, it was the leading provider of customers for European psychiatric hospitals. After many years of infection, the syphilis bacterium can enter the nervous system and cause symptoms such as dementia and 'personality changes'. People go raving mad. There are plenty of famous examples of syphilis causing havoc in the brain, most notably, Prohibition-era gangster Al Capone, who was eventually brought down by his love of brothels. Capone was released from prison on compassionate grounds after beginning to display completely delusional behaviour. He died not long after, at the age of forty-eight.

In 1911, pathologist Peyton Rous made a strange discovery during his studies of chickens with cancer. Rous found that he could transmit the cancer to other chickens using an extract from the cancerous nodule. The cause wasn't cancer cells – or bacteria, for that matter – because it still worked if all cells and bacteria were first filtered out. Instead, the cause turned out to be a virus. It was the first time humans had directly observed a cancer-causing virus.

Rous's attempt didn't attract much interest initially, and it took many years before anyone tried to repeat it. In 1933, other scientists found cancer-causing viruses in rabbits; nine years later, they were found in mice, and then in cats nine years after that. At this point, you can probably guess how the whole thing unfolded. Throughout the period where all these cancer-causing viruses were discovered, there was fierce opposition to the idea that viruses could cause cancer. Especially when some scientists cautiously suggested that there might also be viruses of this kind in humans. As a result, Peyton Rous didn't receive his Nobel Prize until 1966 – fifty-five years after his discovery. This made him the oldest ever Nobel laureate in medicine. Despite the opposition, though, German scientist Harald zur Hausen finally discovered a cancer-causing virus in humans in the 1970s. The virus in question was Human Papillomavirus (HPV), which causes cervical cancer, and which we have previously encountered in the story about Henrietta Lacks. Since then, we have discovered many other cancer-causing viruses in humans. Among them are the Epstein-Barr virus and herpes virus 8, which we have already met, as well as hepatitis B and C, which can cause liver cancer.

Today, we know that about twenty per cent of all cancer cases in humans are caused by microbes. In addition to the many viruses, there are also carcinogenic bacteria, such as our old acquaintance *Helicobacter pylori*, which can cause cancer in the stomach, and *Chlamydia trachomatis* (yes, this time the sexually transmitted disease), which can contribute to cervical cancer alongside HPV. Of all of these, though, HPV is the worst. To be clear, not all HPV viruses are dangerous. There are more than 170 kinds, and most problems arise from the ones called HPV16 and HPV18, which are cancer-causing. The two alone account for about five per cent of *all* cancers in the entire world. The majority of these cases are cervical cancers in women, but we are also seeing an increasing number of men with HPV-caused cancer, including in the oral cavity. This will hopefully be a thing of the past someday, as we have vaccines that can prevent HPV infection (although conspiracy theorists are currently working hard to do the virus's bidding).

Okay, so we know that about twenty per cent of all cancers are caused by microbes. That still leaves the other eighty per cent to have other causes. Maybe. There's still a lot we don't know. In recent years, more and more microorganisms have been found in tumours. It turns out that virtually all tumours in humans are infected by bacteria. That might just be because the cancer suppresses the immune system, making the bacteria take shelter there. But it could also be because the bacteria are helping to form the tumour to begin with. An interesting example is the bacterium *Fusobacterium nucleatum*, which usually lives in the mouth, where it can contribute to cavities in the teeth (again, floss). However, researchers have also found this bacterium in cancers of the colon – and if the tumour spreads, the bacterium follows. Meanwhile, antibiotic treatment to kill the bacterium inhibits growth of the tumour. Similarly, scientists have also found fungi that are 3,000 times more common in tissue samples from pancreases with cancers compared to healthy pancreases.

Exactly how this all ties together is still unclear. Do microbes cause cancer? Do they just promote the growth of cancer? Do microbes help cancer by fighting the immune system? Which are just followers, and which are the culprits? One thing I can say for sure, though, is that the list of cancer-causing microbes is not yet complete.

I think you get the point now. We could continue this chapter with all sorts of other age-related diseases: bacteria from the mouth being found in arterial plaque (floss); influenza increasing the risk of having a heart attack; viruses implicated in the development of Parkinson's disease; and so on and so on. The point is that microbes influence the development of every single age-related disease that plagues us. If we ever want to eradicate these diseases, it will involve fighting against the small critters that prey on us.

★ ★ ★

Imagine for a moment that you're a virus. You're a bit of genetic information in a tiny shell, swimming around in what must feel like an infinite ocean. In reality, it's some poor guy's salivary gland. Your comrades have succeeded in infecting him, and now you're spreading from cell to cell. As with all other biological beings, your ultimate goal is to make a lot of copies of yourself. And for that, you need the molecular apparatus that exists in a cell.

Fortune smiles upon you and you run into a victim. You attach to the surface of the hapless cell and trick it into bringing you inside. Then, your DNA fuses with the cell's own. At that point, it's too late for the cell. If it detects what's happened, it promptly carries out cellular suicide to at least protect the rest of the body. But if this happens, your mission is ruined. You'll lose the opportunity to force the cell to make viral particles. So what do you do? You may remember that one of the triggers for cellular suicide sits on the mitochondria. There are other proteins that can be used to fight viruses here, too, so it's an obvious place for you to attack. You put a brake on the cell's suicide trigger and can breathe a sigh of relief. That doesn't mean you're safe yet, though. The cell is well aware of what's at stake, and has other weapons in its arsenal to deploy against you. If you want to succeed, you have to be quick. The cell is already making viral particles, but you're a greedy little bastard. It should make more, and it should do it fast. So what can you do? You can step on the gas – for example, by mimicking growth signals. Usually, growth means that the cell has to make new cellular components. But if you promote growth now, the extra resources will just be used to make more viral particles. Perfect. All that activity takes energy, though, so you have to be sure that the cell's power plants supply enough. You manipulate the mitochondria some more. By now, the cell is well aware that something is wrong, and it has activated all its stress signals. As you know, stress can trigger autophagy, and infection is no exception. The cell's garbage collectors defend against viruses by collecting viral particles and destroying them. But that's no problem – you just inhibit autophagy so they can't harm you. Gradually, the cell grows desperate. It frantically calls for help from the immune system and tries to warn other nearby cells so they can prepare for virus infection in advance. If the immune system's specialised virus killers find the infected cell, they'll promptly destroy it. And in general, you're just not very fond of these guys. Some immune cells, B-cells, make antibodies, for instance. And antibodies can bind and neutralise specific viruses once an infection is discovered. So in collaboration with your relatives in other infected cells, you take on the immune system, doing everything in your power to deceive it and fight back. As long as that strategy is working, you can continue making more viral particles. Eventually, you'll have produced so many that the cell is completely crammed. Then it's time to move on. You give the cell the death blow by bursting it, so that all the virus particles are released into the infinite ocean in search of the next victim.

Pretty dire, isn't it? Fortunately, no viruses possess *all* these weapons. But just in that little review, we encountered mitochondria, growth signalling, cellular suicide, autophagy, and the immune system. That's a lot of the ageing-related areas we've discussed so far. But in fact the list of ways viruses can impact ageing is even longer. For example:

- Many viruses cause excessive oxidative stress in the cells they infect, just like the oxidative stress we see in older cells.
- Turning into a zombie cell can be a last-minute defence against viruses. The zombie cells 'shut down', and stop dividing, which helps prevent a virus from exploiting the cell.
- Some viruses use the ageing-fighting compound spermidine to make extra copies of themselves. You might remember that we produce less spermidine in old age, and that could be deliberate, as an effort to suppress viruses.
- We've discussed how pathogens sometimes mimic us to escape the immune system. Some take it even further: they mimic our signal molecules. In that way, they try to manipulate us for their own benefit. As an example, we know of viruses that make proteins reminiscent of the growth-promoting hormones IGF-1 and insulin, which are implicated in ageing.

In short, microbes don't just increase the risk of age-related *disease*, they also influence all the things we know play a role in ageing itself. That makes them an even more obvious target for us.

Chapter 17

Immune Rejuvenation

In the ponds of Mozambique and Zimbabwe, there are tiny turquoise fish called killifish. To the untrained eye, they look like ordinary aquarium fish. But when it comes to research on ageing, they're much more than that. Killifish are among the world's shortest-lived vertebrates (animals with a backbone) and they only live a few weeks. This makes them well-suited for studies on ageing because researchers get their results quickly.

Like all other animals, the tiny killifish have microbiomes in their guts, whether they'd like to or not. Actually, many of the bacterial species in the guts of killifish are the same ones living in you and me, making killifish a good model organism for studying gut microbiomes, too. Thus, we arrive at the intersection of gut microbes and ageing.

You see, the ecosystem of the gut changes over time in killifish. As the fish age, they lose diversity in the number of species in the gut, so that a few types of bacteria become dominant while suppressing others. This is exactly the same thing that happens in humans. So scientists in Germany have set out to investigate how these age-related changes in gut bacteria impact ageing and lifespan. The researchers raised killifish until they reached middle-age, and then gave them a course of antibiotics to eradicate the bacteria in their guts. That alone was actually enough to help the fish live longer, but the researchers also wanted to know whether gut bacteria could be beneficial. So, after some of the middle-aged killifish had their gut bacteria wiped out, the scientists recolonised their guts with gut bacteria from young fish. This treatment extended the life of the killifish even further than the antibiotic treatment alone. It seems that certain gut bacteria can help keep us young. But of course, these are the very types of bacteria that we often lose as we age.

Now, I'm not recommending you start popping antibiotics like they're candy. If you do that, you will probably eradicate beneficial bacteria and just improve the odds for harmful ones even more. We might one day have therapies to specifically target those gut bacteria that are causing trouble. But for now, it's worth remembering that the German researchers also found gut bacteria that *helped* the killifish. If we want some of the same effect, it might be worth trying to support these fellows. The bacteria found to be life-extending by the killifish researchers were largely from species that subsist on dietary fibre. These guys are easy to support: just feed them more fibre. In return, they produce a compound called butyrate, which has several health-promoting effects. Among other things, butyrate interacts with the immune system, and it makes the cells lining the gut grip together more tightly. This is important because the intestinal system tends to get leaky as we age. This leakiness means that bacteria from the gut can enter the bloodstream, where they cause trouble – not necessarily because they're *doing* anything, but because our immune system goes crazy. Our immune system reacts strongly to two bacterial molecules called *lipopolysaccharide* (LPS) and *peptidoglycan*. This reaction is helpful if the bacteria is part of some kind of acute infection, but if they're just the result of a passive, low-level stream of microbes into the body, there'll be constant immune activation, and that ends up being harmful.

In general, we see this kind of low-level activation of the immune system a lot in old people. One reason could be an increase in pathogens, but just like everything else in our bodies, the immune system also simply gets worse as we age.

The increased low-level activation of the immune system is called 'chronic inflammation', inflammation being what happens when the immune system is activated. You'll recognise it as warmth, redness, pain and swelling. Not all of this inflammation seems to derive from activation against pathogens. In old people, there is something called 'sterile inflammation', meaning activation of the immune system against no particular enemy. This phenomenon is also called 'inflamm-ageing'. The reason it becomes harmful is because our immune system is not particularly careful. It is evolved to fight infections that used to be life-or-death. So, like soldiers at war, the immune system can't be too concerned about its home. If it manages to kill the bad guys but damages some tissue in the process, that's okay. The alternative could be death.

★ ★ ★

The final piece of the puzzle between microbes and ageing, then, is the immune system itself. We know it starts firing mistakenly in old age. We know it gets worse at fighting pathogens in old age. And we know that many of the genetic variants linked to ageing involve the immune system somehow. But in addition to all this, it seems that an aged immune system in itself promotes ageing. This is illustrated by some research from the University of Minnesota. Here, researchers have created mice in which the immune system ages prematurely. This has all the effects listed above, but it also promotes the ageing of various *other* organs. One reason is that old immune cells can turn into zombie cells, with all the damage that entails. Another is that an ageing and weak immune system fails to remove the other zombie cells that appear in various organs. So, one of the most obvious anti-ageing therapies is actually rejuvenating the immune system.

To achieve immune rejuvenation, researchers target an organ called the thymus. This little organ sits in the chest cavity and is used as a kind of nursery for T-cells – the generals of the immune system. T-cells are made in the bone marrow, but they travel to the thymus to mature. Here, they learn to distinguish self from non-self and finish their development. However, unfortunately, the thymus fares badly during ageing. It undergoes what is called 'thymic involution', where the little organ gradually shrinks and turns into fat. This means we gradually lose our ability to train the generals of the immune system. How fast the thymus diminishes varies between people, but it shrinks between one and three per cent annually in all adults. By the time we reach old age, there's not much left at all.

The decline of the thymus is the number one reason our immune systems get weaker with age. If we could somehow rejuvenate it, it's possible that the rejuvenated immune system would simply fix a lot of the problems we've been discussing in this book. The rejuvenated immune system would clear out zombie cells efficiently. It would be much better at fighting cancer. And it would certainly have no problems with some of the pathogens that haunt old people. Think about how influenza can be harmful in old age but is mostly unproblematic in youth, for instance. In support of this idea, Russian researchers have transplanted thymus tissue from young mice on to old mice. The experiment wasn't particularly pleasant, because the researchers had to transplant the tissue on to the eyes of the poor mice. This is sometimes done because there is low immune activity in the eyes, and thus less risk of losing the graft. But the rather horrifying experiment proved the point, and the young thymus tissue extended the lifespan of the mice.

You probably don't want to replicate the exact experimental set-up described above, but scientists are currently making strides in building 'spare' thymuses from stem cells. The idea is the same as the one we encountered in the section on stem cells – guide stem cells to become cells of the thymus, and then transplant them to people in need. There are proof-of-concept experiments where researchers have made new thymic tissue for mice, so young immune systems in old people might become a reality in the future.

Until then, we actually know at least one method that can potentially halt the decline of the thymus a little. Researchers have managed to partially regenerate the thymus in old mice by giving them zinc supplements. In a clinical trial, other researchers have proved that zinc supplements can also reduce the amount of infections in older people, so maybe the same thing is happening in humans.

Part III
GOOD ADVICE

Chapter 18

Starving for Fun

Imagine we're transported back to Venice in the 1400s. We've gone far enough into the past that the country of Italy doesn't exist yet. Instead, Venice is an independent and incredibly rich city-state. The city produces everything from silk to cotton and glass, and the merchants of Venice distribute exotic goods throughout Europe. Its copious wealth and huge seafaring fleet has made Venice one of Europe's unconditional centres of power.

Among the beautiful canals, we may be lucky enough to encounter a nobleman named Luigi Cornaro. While Cornaro began his life with modest means on the mainland, he later built a fortune by inventing methods for draining wetlands: not a bad occupation in the Venice area.

Cornaro used his fortune to enjoy a life of abundant food and drink, but by the age of forty, this decadent lifestyle had begun to catch up with him. He was overweight, sluggish and feeling old. Ever the innovator, Cornaro decided to take matters into his own hands. And so began a fanatical hunt for a healthier lifestyle.

After consulting with a few doctors, Cornaro came up with a new diet, following a set of strict rules. He'd eat no more than 350g (12¼oz) of food a day, made up of eggs, meat, soup and a little bread. And – naturally, for an Italian – a little wine, too. But only around half a bottle a day.

This new restrictive diet plan worked wonders for Cornaro's health. He was so amazed with his progress that he decided to write a book about his new diet to spread the word. It was, appropriately, titled *Discorsi della vita sobria* – 'Examination of the sober life'.

The book was a huge success and was quickly translated into several other European languages. As for Cornaro himself, he never strayed from the diet again. However, he did continue to experiment, and went on to write several more books on the subject, including *The Art of Living Longer*, which he penned at the age of eighty-three.

By the end of his life, Cornaro had restricted his diet to a single egg yolk at each meal. While not terribly exciting, it seemed to work better than ever. Cornaro was so healthy that he continued his authorship well into his nineties.

When the Grim Reaper finally came knocking on his door, Cornaro had lived the equivalent of two medieval lives, reaching the remarkable age of somewhere between 98 and 102 years old.

★ ★ ★

Nearly four centuries after Luigi Cornaro's death, an American professor was led down the same path as the Venetian nobleman.

Researcher Clive McCay, whom we met while discussing young blood, was a professor at Cornell University in New York State and an expert on nutrition. Back in his time, in the 1930s, there was a lot of focus on helping children grow, preferably as fast as possible, and using vitamins, which were a recent discovery at the time. This zeal for growth worried McCay. He believed that it was better for a person to grow slowly if they wanted to live a long and healthy life.

His inspiration? An English scientist from the sixteenth century with the fitting name of Lord Francis Bacon. Bacon wrote in one of his books exactly what McCay claimed: if you want to live a long life, it is not about growing fast, but about growing as slowly as possible. Preferably to a small adult size. Sound familiar?

To test his theory on growth and longevity, McCay designed an experiment using rats. He divided the rats into three groups. The first group was fed normally, while the other two were fed a diet with significantly fewer calories than normal. McCay made sure the rats weren't malnourished – they got all the vitamins and minerals they needed – just not enough calories. This type of diet has later been named 'calorie restriction'.

As time went on, the rats in the experiment began to die, and McCay attentively noted their lifespans. After 1,200 days, only thirteen of the original 106 rats remained. Every single one of these rats was from one of the calorie-restricted groups. At the time, they had the dubious honour of being the oldest ever laboratory rats.

The rats seemed to prove McCay's theory. Calorie restriction made them grow more slowly, and ultimately end up smaller, while also prolonging their life.

However, decades later, in the 1980s, two scientists, Richard Weindruch and Roy Walford, discovered that growth impediment isn't actually necessary. Calorie restriction still prolongs the life of rodents even if they are allowed to grow to a normal size before their calorie intake is cut down.

Weindruch and Walford also proved that there is a linear relationship between how much you limit calories and how much longer rodents live. Mice fed in abundance live the shortest lives. Mice that are somewhat calorie-restricted live longer. And so it continues until we reach the longest-lived mice of all: those that have been calorie-restricted almost to the point of starvation.

Incidentally, Roy Walford ended up trying calorie restriction on himself.

In 1991, he was part of the first team inside Biosphere 2, the giant futuristic greenhouse, remember? The goal of Biosphere 2 was to create a closed ecosystem that could provide humans and animals with everything needed to sustain life. Walford and his team were locked inside the closed ecosystem for a full two years. As it turns out, building an entire ecosystem from scratch is really hard. The Biosphere 2 team had to drastically cut back their food intake, and eventually required assistance from outside. Over time, it became acceptable to finish each meal by licking the plate clean.

I'm sure you aren't particularly jealous to not have gotten the offer. But for Walford, these conditions were a scoop. His time inside Biosphere 2 allowed him to test calorie restriction on humans and the results were confirmatory. During their famished stay in Biosphere 2, all members of the scientific team had lower blood cholesterol, lower blood pressure, and better immune systems than they'd had before the big experiment.

Since these early studies of calorie restriction, the effect has been proven many times over. When rodents have their calorie intake limited, they typically live between twenty and forty per cent longer than normal. In addition, the animals can reproduce for a longer period of time, have stronger immune systems, are less likely to be affected by cancer and also tend to *look* younger than age-matched controls. However, we know research done in rodents doesn't always translate well to humans (and sometimes not even to other rodents …).

In an effort to get data more applicable to humans, two research groups in the United States have used rhesus monkeys instead of mice or rats. Rhesus monkeys can live for over forty years, so these experiments were a long ordeal. They were started in 1987, and it's only within the last ten years that the results have begun to come out. Were they worth the wait?

When you choose to spend over thirty years on a research project and do precisely two different studies, Murphy's Law dictates that they'll have to give conflicting results. And that's exactly what happened. In the first study, the answer was yes – calorie restriction extended the lifespan of the rhesus monkeys. In fact, one of the monkeys ended up setting the species record for longevity. In the second study, however, there was no particular life extension, although the calorie-restricted monkeys did seem to be healthier while alive.

The conflicting results make it hard to conclusively say whether monkeys fed fewer calories live longer. And we probably shouldn't anticipate that a few million dollars will be set aside for a new experiment with an end date in the middle of the century. So, what can we do to find out if calorie restriction works in humans? It would be pretty difficult, as well as fairly unethical, to do these kinds of studies in humans. Any volunteers to starve?

We do have natural experiments, such as the one from Biosphere 2, of course. And beyond that, there is actually such a thing as calorie-restriction enthusiasts. The 'Calorie Restriction Society' is a group of people who practise voluntary calorie restriction. Of course, humans live even longer than rhesus monkeys, so it's too early to say whether the members of the

Calorie Restriction Society all end up with biblical lifespans. However, studies on these people have shown that their risk parameters for everything from diabetes to cardiovascular disease are absolutely excellent. There's no doubt they are a bunch of unusually healthy people.

Besides these natural experiments, there have also been a few actual trials of calorie restriction. In one example, participants were divided into two groups: group one was told that they should continue to eat normally, while group two was asked to cut their calorie intake by twenty-five per cent over the following two years. Of course, it turned out to be virtually impossible to cut down food intake that much voluntarily. But by the time the two years were over, group two had still managed to reduce their calorie intake by twelve per cent.

Although that's a smaller reduction than planned, it still proved to be enormously beneficial for the participants. Group two members showed improvements across the board. In fact, the changes were reminiscent of those seen in Calorie Restriction Society members, and of the laboratory animals used in calorie restriction research.

Have I convinced you to voluntarily starve? Probably not. For the vast majority of people (including myself), the benefits just aren't great enough.

First, there's the uncertainty – how well will calorie restriction work in humans? In general, it seems that the longer an animal normally lives, the less effectively calorie restriction works. That is, it works great in worms, fine in mice, okay in rhesus monkeys and *maybe* in humans. This is the pattern most life-extension interventions show, actually. I would guess calorie restriction could increase the lifespan of a person by a few years at most – and that's if you know what you're doing.

Second, the reports from the subjects aren't very pleasant. Many report feeling cold, sluggish and fatigued. That's probably how the experimental animals feel, too. Calorie-restricted mice eat like voracious predators if given access to extra food. I guess you could say that it's unsure whether calorie restriction works in people but it will certainly make it *seem* like life is very long.

But while the benefits of calorie restriction may not outweigh the disadvantages, the results of these studies can still be useful to us. For one, they teach us that it's important not to overeat. We might not want to starve ourselves, but there's no reason to eat beyond being full. More importantly, though, we have learned a new strategy for combating ageing. We might not want to employ it as it is, but maybe we can find a way around the drawbacks. Researchers are currently trying to identify ways to mimic the effect of calorie restriction without actually starving. If we can find out exactly *how* calorie restriction affects animals physiologically, we can develop drugs or treatments that mimic the effect.

These kinds of drugs are called calorie restriction mimetics. We've actually met a couple of candidates already: rapamycin and spermidine. But there are also natural ways to replicate the effect of calorie restriction. And that's the second possibility – an approach hidden in wisdom from earlier millennia.

Mechanisms of calorie restriction
There's a lot of research into exactly how calorie restriction works and why it prolongs life. One interesting finding involves the laboratory worm *C. elegans*.

It turns out calorie restriction only extends the lifespan of *C. elegans* if the worms' autophagy, cellular garbage collection system, is functioning. If scientists block autophagy, calorie restriction no longer helps the worms live longer. Another hint pointing in the same direction is that calorie restriction doesn't provide additional benefits in experimental animals on rapamycin. Rapamycin, as you might remember, blocks the growth-promoting mTOR and so activates autophagy.

Chapter 19

An Old Custom in New Clothes

When researchers do calorie restriction experiments, they usually feed their animals once a day. The animals are hungry, so they eat everything at once. Then they fast until the next day. This has led some researchers to suspect that it may be the fasting – and not the reduction in calorie intake – that is responsible for prolonging life. In an ingenious experiment that supports this idea, researchers put mice on calorie restriction in a different way. Instead of giving the mice small amounts of typical food, they were given a special kind of chow with a very low calorie content. The mice were allowed to eat all day – and they did – but they still ended up getting limited calories. In this way, the researchers created calorie restriction without fasting. Now, if eating fewer calories is what is beneficial to the mice, these mice should still have had prolonged lifespans. However, if *fasting* is actually the cause of life extension, the mice *wouldn't* live longer, as they were eating throughout the day. The result was the latter: when mice are calorie-restricted without fasting, they don't live longer than usual.

Other researchers have attacked the question from the opposite angle: they have made mice fast while not reducing their overall food intake. This can be done by only feeding the mice every other day. The mice will typically eat twice as much as usual on the days they are fed, so they don't get fewer calories than normal, but they are fasting in between. And that is enough to prolong their life. In fact, their fasted mice live almost as long as calorie-restricted mice.

At this point, there is little doubt that fasting can mimic the effect of calorie restriction and extend lifespan in rodents. It makes good sense, too, and fits in with our previous discoveries. For example, fasting is a kind of hormesis: a stressor that ultimately makes us stronger. And just like calorie restriction, fasting also inhibits the growth promoter mTOR while increasing the activity of the cellular garbage collectors, autophagy.

★ ★ ★

Fasting is a widespread phenomenon in most of the world. We see it in nearly every culture and religion. As far back as ancient Greece, Hippocrates – the father of modern medicine – recommended fasting for health-related reasons. And the historian Plutarch, who lived a few hundred years later, said: 'Fast today instead of using medicine.' To this day, fasting is part of all the major world religions. Orthodox Christians have fasting periods, including the forty days between Shrove Tuesday and Easter; Jews have regular fast days, including the holiest day, Yom Kippur, where you don't eat from sundown one day until sundown the next day; Muslims celebrate the annual month of Ramadan, where neither food nor drink is allowed while the sun is up; Buddhists fast during periods of intense meditation; and Hindus too have a wide variety of fasts throughout the year. In fact, fasting is so common that you'd be hard pressed to find a culture or religion that doesn't have a fasting tradition of some sort.

Now, of course, these religions don't prescribe fasting to fight ageing, but religious texts *do* frequently describe fasting as something healthy. Whether it is about cleansing (autophagy?), strength through trials (hormesis?), mental clarity or self-reflection.

Fasting is implemented in a variety of different ways as well. Some people don't eat anything at all, some just omit certain kinds of foods (especially meat), some eat much less than usual, and some refrain from eating during particular times.

Similarly, there are almost as many research-based ways of fasting as there are religious ones. Let's take a look. A common way to fast is to restrict your eating window, which is known as time-restricted feeding. We all do this to some extent. Unless you're one of those people who snack late at night or get up in the middle of the night to do it, you fast from dinner one day to breakfast the next. Some people experiment with extending this fasting period, for example by eating all their food within a window of four to eight hours, instead of the typical twelve to fourteen hours.

This approach has had some promising results in mice. For instance, studies show that time-restricted eating protects mice from the negative effects of an unhealthy diet, whether that diet is high in sugar or high in fat. To put it another way, in mice an unhealthy diet can – to some extent – be neutralised by time-restricted eating. I can imagine using a similar strategy during the holidays which is, in fact, the time period where people tend to put on most weight.

Beyond time-restricted eating, most other fasting methods involve undertaking all-day fasts for one or more days. This type of fasting is known as intermittent fasting, and is the kind of fasting we particularly see in religious texts.

The scientific history of intermittent fasting originated in the 1940s with the researchers Anton Carlson and Frederick Hoelzel of the University of Chicago. The two were something of an odd couple. Carlson was an eminent Swedish-American physiologist with a PhD from Stanford University who chaired the Department of Physiology at the University of Chicago for twenty-four years.

Hoelzel also ended up as a researcher, though his path there was a little more curious. As a teenager, he'd developed terrible stomach pains, and nothing made them go away. Eventually, he became convinced that the pain was caused by the food he was eating. His solution was simple: just don't eat anything. That turned out to be too hard, so instead Hoelzel started eating 'alternative' foods to keep his hunger under control. He tried, among other things, coal, sand, hair, feathers and – his favourite – surgical cotton.

After Carlson and Hoelzel's paths crossed, they became friends and ended up as a dynamic scientific duo. When they weren't testing the passage time of the various objects Hoelzel ate (glass balls passed faster than gold flakes, for example), they also tested more legitimate physiological questions together.

In 1946, they carried out what is now a famous experiment involving fasting and mice. The two were inspired by Clive McCay's study on life extension using calorie restriction. They thought, quite reasonably, that it wouldn't be possible to carry over that method to humans in a pleasant way. Instead, they argued, inspiration should be drawn from the only similar phenomenon in the real world: religious fasting.

They tested that idea and found that, yes indeed, periodic fasting was beneficial for rats in an experimental setting. Carlson and Hoelzel's results added this kind of fasting to the – at the time – very short list of ways to extend the life of rats.

The method Carlson and Hoelzel used on their rats is called alternate-day fasting, an approach that involves fasting every other day and otherwise eating normally. Today, it has become a popular method in health circles and among people who want to lose weight. The method is quite simple: days of fasting are alternated with days of eating normally to satiety. Some people don't fast entirely, but eat a small amount of food, for example 500–600 calories, to keep hunger at bay. A slightly gentler alternative is the 5:2 diet, which is also popular. The principles are like those of alternate-day fasting, but you only fast for two days a week.

We're still collecting evidence of the effects of intermittent fasting in humans. One caveat when translating the mouse studies to humans is that a whole day of fasting is a lot longer for a mouse than a person. A mouse lives a few years at best, while humans live for decades. So some scientists think we will have to undertake longer fasts to get the same benefits as the laboratory mice.

One of the proponents of longer fasts is the renowned researcher Valter Longo. Longo and his colleagues found that many of the beneficial effects of a fast only appear after three days. The problem with that, of course, is that fasting for three days is not very pleasant or convenient, especially if you have a normal life that needs to be held together (and there are probably very few people who want to spend their vacations or weekends fasting).

The solution Longo and his colleagues have come up with is the so-called fasting-mimicking diet which they envision healthy people occasionally using. As the name suggests, this diet simulates a complete fast without actually being one. The fast lasts five days, in which participants eat very small meals with a low calorie content. The meals are high in fat and are designed to trick the body into thinking that it is fasting because that normally involves burning our own body fat for fuel.

★ ★ ★

Some people might get nervous at the thought of longer fasts, and not without reason. Obviously, there are people who shouldn't fast for long periods, like children, pregnant women, sick people and the elderly. But for healthy adults, fasting for a few days is fine, as long as you remember to drink plenty of water. The general rule is that humans can survive three minutes without oxygen, three days without water and three weeks without food. But the last one isn't always accurate; if you have enough fat for your body to burn, you can go significantly longer.

The world record for the longest fast is held by the Scotsman Angus Barbieri. As a twenty-seven-year-old, Barbieri weighed 207kg (456lb). He knew that he was facing an early death and desperately wanted to lose weight. Back then, in the 1960s, there was a lot of research into using fasting for weight loss. The logic was basically that you should stop eating until you reached your desired weight.

Barbieri was willing to give fasting a try, so he showed up at Maryfield Hospital in Dundee near his hometown. He told doctors he was ready to give up food to lose weight and feeling his determination, the doctors agreed to monitor Barbieri while he fasted.

To begin with, Barbieri hadn't planned to fast for anything more than a short period of time. But as time went on, he became more and more focused on reaching his ideal weight. Doctors agreed to let him continue, but started giving him a multivitamin pill to make sure he didn't become deficient in anything. Besides that, though, the heavily overweight Barbieri didn't need much – his body had enough fuel to sustain itself.

Weeks turned into months as Barbieri stubbornly chased his ideal weight of 82kg (181lb). When he finally reached his goal, he had been fasting for *382 days*. That's a year and seventeen days without eating. Incredibly, Barbieri managed to maintain his weight loss. When the doctors caught up with him again five years later, he'd put on only 7kg (15lb).

A fast of that duration obviously *isn't* something that I'd recommend for anyone, no matter how overweight they might be. The reason we don't use Barbieri's method today is that some people who attempted it after him ended up dying.

In addition to the safety issue, the most common objection to fasting is that you go into a state of starvation and begin to break down muscles if you do not eat constantly. It is true that if you fast for a long time, your body slows down your metabolism and will eventually start burning muscle for fuel. However, this isn't something that would happen during a day or two of fasting. Studies show that metabolism doesn't decrease if, for example, a person fasts every other day. In fact, metabolism and fat burning increases. This makes sense evolutionarily; when an animal lacks food, it must go out to find it, and this means that its activity should increase, not decrease.

In addition, research shows that people who start strength training and, at the same time, eat within a restricted window gain the same amount of muscle mass as people who eat regularly. And in one study where subjects fasted every other day for eight weeks, their fat mass dropped, but their muscle mass didn't.

Feel free to have another cup of coffee

Studies suggest that people who drink a few cups of coffee a day (between two and four) have a lower mortality rate than those who don't drink coffee at all. Now, this doesn't mean the coffee drinking *causes* this difference, but there are some aspects of coffee that we could at least imagine to be beneficial. For one, caffeine is an appetite suppressant, and we know eating less can be beneficial. Some people even use coffee when fasting, as it can help keep hunger at bay and is calorie-free when no milk, sugar or cream is added. However, even drinking decaf coffee is correlated to a longer life, so it is possible the health benefits of coffee comes from something else as well.

Chapter 20

Cargo Cult Nutrition

Calorie restriction might be a good life-extension strategy, but at some point we *do* have to eat. The question is: eat what?

There are so many different diets out there that we could experiment for the rest of our lives: low-carb or low-fat? How about going vegan? Or perhaps trying the Paleo diet, the ketogenic diet, the Mediterranean diet or maybe the gummy bear diet?

When you first start looking into nutrition, it's easy to pick a new diet with confidence. You'll encounter a credible-sounding guru and he'll tell you something surprising. Bacon is actually healthy! And here's a study to back it up. The study will be legitimate, with nice graphs and fancy-sounding words. You see, says the guru, everyone else is ignorant. There's no need to worry, my data clearly shows bacon is healthy.

One day, as you're munching down a tray of bacon while arguing with your family members, you look up that homerun of a study again. That'll teach them! But in the process, you find another study. This one concludes the opposite – bacon *is* going to give you a heart attack. The study has many references supporting it, and at the bottom of the rabbit hole is another credible-sounding guru. He matter-of-factly explains that bacon is the *number one* bad food, and anyone consuming it will die an early death. You push the tray aside. How could you have been so stupid?

Months pass, and one night while reading the news, you stumble on an article. 'New study: Bacon might increase your lifespan.' The article interviews yet another credible-sounding guru. He explains why old studies on bacon are fundamentally flawed. His new study, which corrects these flaws, proves bacon is supremely healthy. 'I was sceptical at first,' he says. But after going on an all-bacon diet, he has lost 100lb and can now bench-press a small family sedan.

Alright, while I might exaggerate a little, the world of nutrition science really is notoriously hard to navigate. The same foods will be healthy one day, then unhealthy the next – or maybe both at once – according to different sources. And it doesn't take much digging before every food seems like it's going to give you cancer.

There are a whole bunch of reasons why nutrition science is so contradictory. An obvious one is that some studies are funded by food companies. To everyone's surprise, it turns out industry-sponsored studies often yield results that are beneficial to their donors.

In other cases, however, evil food companies are not to blame. Sometimes *we* are. A study claiming that chocolate is actually healthy will be celebrated on the rooftops. Meanwhile, the twenty contradicting studies will be forgotten. It's a lot easier to convince people of something that is convenient or pleasurable; our rationalising brain will grasp at any opportunity to justify eating more chocolate. But as the famous physicist Richard Feynman said: 'The first principle is that you must not fool yourself – and you are the easiest person to fool.'

Alongside these obvious problems, however, there are also some more subtle issues that we need to be aware of if we want to eat our way to a long life.

* * *

During the Second World War, the American and Japanese militaries built airbases on several South Pacific islands. The bases provided many native islanders with their first face-to-face encounters with the modern world. They were astonished. Here they were, toiling for everything they had – attending to their crops and livestock, building houses and making weapons by hand. Meanwhile, the foreigners had an endless supply of food, clothes, medicine and otherworldly equipment supplied to them from above. They would perform a few rituals, like marching back and forth, yelling at each other and waving at the sky. Then huge machines would appear, carrying more goods than the natives could produce in several lifetimes. Only the gods could be powerful enough to be the source of this abundance.

Eventually, though, the war ended, the foreigners disappeared – and so did all their precious cargo. The natives desperately wanted the planes to return. But how? They tried turning to the gods, imitating the strange rituals of the foreigners. They cleared airstrips in the forest and marched up and down them with bamboo guns. They made headsets and radios from coco-nuts and straws. They even built wooden offices, air control towers and airplanes. Eventually, the whole thing turned into several religions dubbed 'cargo cults' by anthropologists. Some of these cargo cults still exist today, believing that, one day, the gods will notice their rituals and start sending cargo planes once again.

The members of the cargo cults employ one of our most powerful learning techniques: imitation of successful people. In our world, you might copy everything about your favourite sports star, musician or business person. It's not always obvious what causes these people to be successful, so if you want similar success, it makes sense to copy pretty much everything – whether that's starting your day at 4 a.m. with an ice bath, reading voraciously, or only wearing black turtlenecks. However, when we're not aware of the 'generator' of success, we risk just copying a bunch of insignificant surface-level features like the cargo cults.

Something similar actually happens all the time in nutrition science. We study long-lived people, trying to uncover the secrets of longevity, but often we simply end up copying a bunch of the surface-level features of rich, educated people. You see, on average, rich, educated people live longer than poor, less-educated people. Someone with a bachelor's degree can expect to live several years longer than someone with only a high school degree. This trend holds true in every country around the world and the gap seems to be growing over time.

This longevity gap is due to the fact that wealth and education make people follow health guidelines more closely. Why that is, I will leave up to sociologists. But the facts are that the wealthier and more educated you are, the more likely you are to exercise regularly, get vaccinated, be a non-smoker and have a healthy body weight. These health-promoting habits are obviously great to copy, but how do we separate them from everything else that rich, educated people are up to?

For instance, we know wearing glasses is more common among educated groups of people. If we made a study trying to find traits that correlate with living a long life, wearing glasses would thus be one of them. But the fact that someone wears glasses obviously doesn't affect their lifespan. We couldn't pick some guy off the street and prolong his life by putting a pair of glasses on him. Nor would I advise you to intentionally ruin your vision in a quest for longevity.

You might have heard the phrase 'correlation doesn't imply causation'. Essentially, two things can be correlated (even tightly) without one causing the other. The natives of the South Pacific observed that there was a tight correlation between making gestures towards the sky and the arrival of an airplane. But these gestures had nothing to do with *causing* the airplane to arrive. Similarly, there's a strong correlation between how many people die of heatstroke on a given day and how much ice cream is sold. However, that doesn't mean eating ice cream makes people get heat stroke and die. Instead, both ice cream sales and the number of heat strokes are caused by hotter temperatures, and do not affect each other whatsoever.

There's a real-life example of a longevity cargo cult arising from the sunny town of Loma Linda in southern California. Loma Linda is known as one of the Blue Zones, and its inhabitants have been studied extensively for their longevity. Many Loma Lindans are Seventh-Day Adventists and abstain from eating meat due to their religion (originally inspired by John Harvey Kellogg, whose breakfast products you might have tried). After decades of research, the consensus is that a meatless lifestyle yields approximately three additional years of life. In Loma Linda, the vegans live the longest, then the vegetarians, followed by semi-vegetarians and finally the meat-eaters.

But as you might've guessed, there's more to the numbers. Veganism and vegetarianism are mostly popular among rich, educated people. You'll see a lot more plant-based restaurants in a university town than in a trailer park. That means vegans and vegetarians tend to have lots of other healthy habits: they exercise more than average, drink less alcohol, smoke less and have healthier body weights. Mirroring their lifespans, the vegans of Loma Linda have an average BMI of 23. The vegetarians have one of 25.5. The semi-vegetarians have a BMI of 27, while for the meat-eaters the average is 28. So is it really the lack of meat that prolongs life?

Epidemiologists are well aware of the problem, and have devised several potential solutions. The most common one is to try to account for health differences before comparing groups of people. For instance, before comparing the lifespans of vegans and meat-eaters, we could subtract the effect we know comes from extra exercise, less smoking and healthier BMIs among vegans. In this way, we can pretend we're comparing similar groups of people. Once you actually do this, veganism no longer extends life.

Another good example is red wine. There are lots of studies claiming red wine will make you live longer because red-wine drinking and longevity are correlated. Studies have been busy trying to find the source of the health benefits and ascribed them to all sorts of molecules found in red wine. But to no one's surprise, red wine is disproportionally favoured by rich, educated people. That means people who drink a lot of red wine are like the vegans and vegetarians discussed above. They have lower than average BMIs as well as generally healthy habits, so we cannot conclude that red wine is making these people healthy. It is most likely all their other habits.

★ ★ ★

If we really want to know if a food or habit is not just *correlated* with health benefits but actually *causes* them, the gold standard is something called a randomised controlled trial. We've encountered the concept a few times already. In a randomised controlled trial, scientists gather together a bunch of people and divide them into two groups with equal baseline characteristics. One group is given an intervention – a drug, a new exercise routine, a new diet – while the other group is given placebo. Then, time is allowed to pass to see whether there is a disparity in a certain outcome, such as lifespan or the development of a disease.

For instance, we might have noticed that people eating a lot of spinach tend to have big muscles. If we want to learn whether spinach *causes* your muscles to grow, we could do a randomised controlled trial. Here, we would gather test subjects, divide them into two groups and ask one group to eat spinach every day for the following months. Then we would track whether this group had increased muscle growth compared to the other group who continued as normal.

While randomised controlled trials are harder to do than simply looking for correlations, you'd be surprised just how many things have been investigated this way throughout the years. We're talking stuff like using live parasites to cure allergies, or fighting blindness using proteins from algae. However, modern medicine also has its favourites. In particular, there are two supplements that have been tested in randomised controlled trials for practically *everything* – and that includes their ability to prolong life.

The first one is fish oil – or more specifically, omega-3 fatty acids. Omega-3s are polyunsaturated fatty acids that serve vital roles in our physiology. Among other things, we use them in cellular membranes and as a starting material for making other important compounds. We mostly get omega-3s from our food, and the best dietary source is fatty fish such as salmon, mackerel and herring. Research has repeatedly found that a high fish consumption is associated with living a long life, and omega-3s are the main suspect. For instance, the more omega-3 fatty acids someone has in their blood or cellular membranes, the longer they tend to live.

At this point, your new bullshit filter might be springing into action. Don't rich, educated people eat more fish than others? Is that the reason for these correlations? There are certainly more seafood dishes at fancy restaurants than at McDonald's. Health authorities have been recommending fish for decades, and studies do indeed show that rich, educated people eat the most fish. That's why we should skip the correlations and turn to randomised controlled trials instead.

In randomised controlled trials for fish oil, the health benefits are much more modest than we might have naively expected. It turns out, much of the correlation between fish consumption and health *is* due to rich, educated people eating more fish, rather than anything to do with fish itself. However, to be fair, the health benefits are not totally gone. If we put on our rose-coloured glasses and squint a little, randomised controlled trials show that fish oil supplements could have a few health benefits. They particularly seem to lower the risk of various diseases of the heart and cardiovascular systems, working better at high doses.

So given that fish is tasty and fish oil supplements are easy to take, it can't hurt to include them in a longevity conscious diet. There are no indications of harm in the millions of people studied, meaning the worst that can happen is you experience no benefits. As always, it is preferable to eat the food itself rather than take a supplement. Fish might have other health-promoting effects beyond those obtainable from fish oil. But fish is also expensive and frankly – if you're anything like me – hard to cook.

When using fish oil supplements, it's important to pick one that has been tested for omega-3 content. Some contain very little, while others might contain pollutants or be of poor quality. There's a lot of fraud out there.

There's even fraud going on with *actual* fish and seafood. In a number of tragicomical studies, scientists have found that a lot of fish sold in restaurants and supermarkets is not what it claims to be. Someone, somewhere in the supply chain must have reasoned that people don't know anything about fish. Then they've straight-up replaced fancy fish with something cheaper. For instance, in a study done in several countries, forty per cent of 'snapper' on sale was found to not actually be snapper at all. In another study, up to half of the sushi tested in Los Angeles was made with a different fish than claimed. And in a third study, many 'prawn balls' in Singapore didn't contain any prawns at all. Someone managed to replace it with *pork* and get away with it.

★ ★ ★

If fish oil is the prince of supplements, then vitamin D is the king. There are so many vitamin D studies out there that frankly you should feel sorry for me for having to review them.

Once again, the surface-level story is perfectly clear. Low vitamin D levels are robustly associated with dying early. However, as I've been repeating to the point of madness now, that doesn't necessarily mean that there is causation. Actually, there are a bunch of reasons to believe there is *no* causation.

First, we might have the whole thing backwards. It turns out that many diseases cause vitamin D levels to drop – not the other way around. That means low vitamin D levels don't cause the diseases it has been linked to. Instead *the diseases* are what cause the low vitamin D levels.

Second, there is our pet peeve issue that poor people tend to have lower vitamin D levels than wealthy people.

And third, vitamin D is a fat-soluble vitamin (or actually a hormone). It seems people with excess fat mass have low vitamin D levels, and this could be because of entrapment in fat tissue. In other words, being overweight might make your vitamin D levels lower, and we know excess weight also promotes the development of several diseases.

To figure out this chicken-and-egg situation, we must once again turn to randomised controlled trials. That is, studies where scientists give people vitamin D supplements and follow them to uncover whether it improves their health.

In the case of vitamin D, we *really* have to put on rose-coloured glasses to find a benefit. When pooling the many studies together, scientists find that vitamin D supplements do not decrease your risk of dying or your risk of the most important age-related diseases. For the sake of longevity, you can use your money on something else.

Is alcohol bad?

There's no doubt that it's extremely unhealthy to drink too much alcohol. The big health question, though, is whether it's beneficial – or at least okay – to have a few drinks. In correlational studies between alcohol intake and longevity, there is a J-shaped curve that looks like hormesis. That is,

---

people who drink a little alcohol actually live longer than those who don't drink at all (while those that drink a lot obviously die earlier than both). The fact that light drinking extends lifespan is one of those beliefs that it is easy to convince yourself of. After all, that would be nice, wouldn't it? As a result, the health benefits of a little alcohol are oft-touted. But of course, that also means scepticism is warranted.

The problem with these studies is that the group of people who don't drink at all includes many former alcoholics. Years of alcohol abuse will cause lasting damage, so even if an alcoholic has managed to quit drinking, their life expectancy is still reduced (though far less than if they had continued). As a result, the group of 'non-drinkers' are a patchwork of lifelong teetotallers and former alcoholics. And if you remove the former alcoholics, the benefits of a few drinks a week disappear – light drinkers don't live longer than teetotallers after all. However, to be fair, there's still not a huge amount of difference between teetotallers and light drinkers as long as it entails staying below five drinks a week.

Chapter 21

Food for Thought

The enzyme amylase is an important part of our carbohydrate metabolism. We secrete amylase in our saliva and digestive system, where it helps us break down starch from foods such as bread, rice and potatoes. This means amylase is especially important to someone eating an agricultural diet. When hunter-gatherers settled down and started farming, one's ability to digest starch became vital to health and survival. We can see the shadow of this in our genetics today.

You see, humans have evolved to have multiple copies of the amylase gene (and interestingly, so have our dogs). All the copies do the same thing – make amylase – but having multiple copies helps us make more and improves starch digestion.

Our switch to farming happened relatively recently on the evolutionary timescales, and at different times across the world. This means adaptations to agricultural diets are not yet universally distributed. For instance, scientists have found that the number of amylase genes varies from two copies in some people to more than ten in others. On average, people from populations that have farmed for a long time, such as Europeans and East Asians, have more amylase genes than agricultural latecomers. However, even among Europeans and East

Asians, some individuals have few amylase genes, making them less well-suited to a high-starch diet.

Amylase is just a minor component of our metabolism, but we know of several other genetic variants that are similarly skewed in their distribution. A classic example is genetic variants that allow one to break down lactose, the sugar found in milk. Originally, only infants could digest lactose, which was needed to enable them to subsist on breast milk. However, thousands of years ago, mutations arose extending this ability into adulthood. Such mutations would be useless to hunter-gatherers (where would they get the milk?) but to a farmer who can now subsist on dairy, they are pure gold. In my native Denmark – close to the origin of these mutations – almost every adult can digest lactose today. The mutations become rarer as you move away from Northern Europe, but that's just because they haven't had the time to spread yet. It's an obvious advantage to a farmer to be lactose tolerant. If we hadn't reached modernity lactose tolerance would continue spreading because those able to digest milk could get more calories and increase their chance at surviving and having children. For now, though, lactose tolerance is unequally distributed, and the exact same food can be a healthy source of calcium for some while giving other people explosive diarrhoea.

In some instances, there are even *opposing* genetic variants in different people. Take the genes FADS1 and FADS2, which encode enzymes involved in the body's production of molecules called long-chain polyunsaturated fatty acids. Among these tongue-twisting molecules are some omega-3 fatty acids. The Inuit people of Greenland have eaten fish-heavy diets for thousands of years, which provide them with omega-3s in abundance. As a result, they have high frequencies of genetic variants in FADS1 and FADS2, which limits the body's own production because it's just not needed when the molecules are easily obtainable from the diet. On the other hand, there are historically vegetarian communities in Pune, India, where most people have versions of FADS2 that *improve* their body's production of long-chain polyunsaturated fatty acids. This is strongly advantageous when dietary intake is low, as it is on a vegetarian diet.

So, should you eat a low-carb diet for health? Drink milk? Go vegetarian? The piece of the puzzle we've been missing so far is that the answer depends on your genetics. One of your friends might try a vegetarian diet and fare brilliantly, while you feel better on a low-carb diet. That doesn't necessarily mean one of you is lying, or that one of you is healthier than the other, even though your diets are almost completely inverted.

★ ★ ★

Most of our health efforts are still performed somewhat blindly. We hear something is 'healthy' and then cross our fingers that it's true. As you might have learned by now, a lot of the time it isn't. Something can be healthy for you without being healthy for me. For instance, when a study concludes: 'Muscle mass was increased twenty-five per cent by eating spinach,' that is true *on average*. But that doesn't mean every single person who ate spinach gained twenty-five per cent more muscle mass. Some gained more, some gained less; some might have gained none at all or even lost muscle mass. As we've learned, we're not always comparable and that's why the blind approach often fails. So instead of guessing, we should actually measure what is going on in our bodies and tailor our approach accordingly. For instance, we could start eating spinach and actually measure how it affects our own muscle mass, strength or bio-markers of the blood. Or we could use combinations of these measurements to pick the optimal diet, exercise routine or lifestyle.

The reason we're not already collecting data about ourselves at scale like this comes down to technological and economical limitations. In some cases, we lack knowledge – for instance, when it comes to interpreting a lot of our genetics. We can 'read' our genes using what is called 'genome sequencing', but the interpretation is harder and still at the early stages.

In other cases, we know what to do, but it is troublesome. For instance, we still need invasive blood draws to measure most biomarkers of the blood, such as hormone levels, metab-olites, vitamins and markers of inflammation. In most cases, it is too expensive to measure biomarkers frequently. If you have any expertise or interest in these areas, you hereby have my strongest recommendation to give it a shot and help us all out. Gaining access to more data about our bodies could unlock a revolution in health and wellness.

As we've discussed already, the holy grail of biomarkers for longevity is an accurate biological clock. That is, some biomarker we can track over time to determine the rate at which our bodies are ageing. The best bets are currently telomere-shortening and epigenetic clocks. Both are useful when studying large groups of people, but unfortunately biological clocks are not precise enough to be accurate for individuals – yet.

For now, the smart choice is to use the biomarkers that are readily available to us. An obvious one is body weight, as it is well known being overweight or obese comes with significant health drawbacks. However, there are also biomarkers of the blood worth investigating, though they still require a doctor's appointment. Let's take a look.

Chapter 22

Medieval Monks to Modern Science

As we've discussed previously, one of the best ways to prolong the life of the tiny worm *C. elegans* is to disable the worm's version of the growth-promoting gene IGF-1. The actual name of this gene is daf-2, and it is not just a stand-in for IGF-1 – it's also the worm's version of the hormone insulin.

Insulin, like IGF-1, is growth-promoting, but its primary role is to regulate blood sugar. When we eat carbohydrates, enzymes in the gut break down most of the various forms into the simple sugar glucose. We absorb this glucose, and after entering the blood it is called 'blood sugar'. Our cells use sugar from the blood as fuel, and this is where insulin comes into the picture. When our blood sugar rises after a meal, we secrete insulin from the pancreas to enable cellular uptake. You can imagine insulin as a tiny key that opens a gate in the cell, allowing sugar to enter. This mechanism helps us fuel our cells, but it is also necessary because high blood sugar levels can damage our blood vessels. This means we want to lower blood sugar when it spikes after eating, even if our cells don't need energy at the time. We primarily do so by shuttling the sugar to fat cells, where it can be converted into fat and stored. If blood sugar levels still remain high, though, the last resort is to excrete it in our urine.

Since ancient Egyptian times, doctors have described patients with endless thirst, fatigue and a tendency to urinate a lot. For some reason, multiple people have discovered that the urine of these patients tends to taste sweet. We now know this is because the patients' bodies are trying to lower their blood sugar. They have diabetes, known as 'sugar sickness' in my native Danish. In diabetes, insulin fails to lower blood sugar sufficiently, making the body desperate to get rid of it. There's an autoimmune version, type 1 diabetes, where the immune system mistakenly kills the insulin-producing cells. But there's also a lifestyle-dependent version called type 2 diabetes. Here, patients do produce insulin, but their cells become ever less responsive to it. The key stops being able to open the gate. This especially seems to happen to over-weight people and people who eat high amounts of pro-cessed foods.

While type 2 diabetes is a disease, there are actually levels of what is called 'insulin sensitivity' even among healthy people. That is, different people require different amounts of insulin to remove sugar from the blood. You can imagine insulin sen-sitivity as a spectrum. At one end, the cells of an athlete will be insulin sensitive, requiring only a small amount of insulin to take up blood sugar. At the other end, the cells of a diabetic person will not react even at high insulin levels.

If we extrapolate from the worm *C. elegans*, insulin-sensitive people should live longer. After all, dampening the equivalent of insulin signalling increases the lifespan of the worms. Scien-tists find that human centenarians do indeed tend to be insu-lin sensitive and have tight blood sugar control. Similarly, the lifespan of mice can be increased by disabling insulin signalling in fat cells.

Unfortunately, insulin and blood sugar levels tend to rise with age, and so does the risk of diabetes. In the 1990s, Swedish researcher Staffan Lindeberg wondered whether it really has to be this way. Lindeberg was studying the people of Kitava, a lush tropical island belonging to Papua New Guinea. The traditional diet of the Kitavans is based on local crops, such as yams, taro, fruit and coconuts, supplemented with a little fish. This diet is sixty-nine per cent carbohydrates, or high-carb if you will. We might naively expect that to mean the Kitavans would tend to have high blood sugar and insulin levels.

Lindeberg tested this theory by collecting blood samples from average Swedes and comparing them to blood samples from the Kitavans. He found that the Kitavans had less insulin in their blood than Swedes, despite eating a more carbohydrate-rich diet. And while insulin levels rose with age among the Swedes, there was no such increase among the Kitavans. In general, the Kitavans were exceptionally healthy. Lindeberg only managed to find two overweight people on the island and both were just back home visiting after having moved to a big city on the mainland to become businessmen.

The Kitavans prove that carbohydrates per se are not the problem when it comes to insulin sensitivity. If you have a healthy weight, like the Kitavans, and your carbohydrates are whole foods, not candy, you'll be insulin sensitive and healthy. However, realistically, most of us will not be able to eat like the Kitavans all the time. If we still want to be healthy, the optimal approach would be to measure our insulin sensitivity and blood sugar levels while experimenting with different diets or foods. We know that people can have very different-sized blood sugar spikes upon eating the same foods, from oatmeal to candy. Some of that could be due to genetics, but another reason is the gut microbiome. There is a curious correlation between specific species of gut bacteria and the size of blood-glucose spikes from different foods.

The less time-consuming and equipment-heavy approach to becoming more like the Kitavans would be to adopt some tried-and-true habits. The best one is to exercise – or just move – after eating. The muscles are the primary destination for blood sugar, and the simple act of using them can help lower blood sugar spikes substantially. Even a short walk or some bodyweight movements after a meal can be beneficial.

There are, however, also more drastic approaches to taming blood sugar, the most fascinating of which takes us to the gardens of medieval monasteries.

★ ★ ★

If you were living in the Middle Ages and began feeling symptoms of diabetes, such as unquenchable thirst, fatigue and frequent urination, you might get sent to some monk at a monastery. Upon listening to your complaints, he would go to the garden, pick up a beautiful purple shrub and grind up a preparation for you. The shrub – French lilac, or goat's rue – is not some hocus-pocus treatment. A substance from this perennial can actually lower blood sugar and mitigate symptoms of diabetes. We still use it today, although the original substance has been further developed into a drug. This drug is called metformin and it was approved for the treatment of diabetes in 1957. Since then, it has been one of the most widely used diabetes medications worldwide.

After spending decades as an anonymous diabetes drug, metformin has suddenly burst on to the anti-ageing stage. In a now-famous study, researchers compared the lifespans of three groups: healthy people, diabetics on metformin and diabetics using other drugs. As expected, most diabetics lived shorter lives than average. Save one glaring exception: diabetics on metformin lived *longer* than the non-diabetic average. That is, when using metformin, these people – who are suffering from a life-shortening disease – lived longer than comparable healthy controls. Does that mean metformin is the first anti-ageing drug?

It might surprise you to learn that while we know the *effects* of metformin – lowered blood sugar, improved insulin sensitivity – we don't actually know *how* it works, even though it was approved decades ago and is used daily by millions of people. The most widely accepted theory is that metformin activates an enzyme called AMPK which works like an energy sensor in our cells. Under normal conditions, AMPK is activated when the cell lacks energy. It switches the cell into a kind of energy-saving state, as seen when a person is fasting or on a calorie-restrictive diet. Metformin advocates argue this makes metformin like fasting in pill form.

A second theory is that metformin doesn't actually work on *us*, but on our gut bacteria. Giving mice metformin improves their insulin sensitivity, but you can transfer the effect by transferring the gut bacteria. That is, by taking the gut bacteria from a metformin-treated mouse and giving it to a new mouse, the new mouse also becomes more insulin sensitive, even if it never got the drug itself. Both effects could be right and contribute independently. It is not uncommon for drugs to work in several different places at once. Actually, our bodies are so complex that it's nearly impossible to make a drug that *won't* impact us in multiple ways. When initially designing drugs, researchers simply cross their fingers that none of these extra interactions will lead to unwanted side effects.

A third theory about metformin is that it inhibits inflammation, and this is where it runs into trouble in my opinion. Inhibiting inflammation in the body might sound like a good thing, but you have to remember that inflammation – and damage in general – is not always bad. Sure, if you have high levels of inflammation because you live on chips and soda, it may be a good idea to alleviate it. But inflammation is also a key player in hormesis. For instance, after exercise, there are heightened levels of inflammation that serve as one of the 'damage signals' that initiate a cascade of healthy adaptations. So by inhibiting inflammation, metformin seems to also inhibit the beneficial effects of exercise. When people who don't usually exercise take metformin and start training, they don't gain as much endurance or muscle mass as those who don't take metformin and they also miss out on key cellular adaptations to exercise.

That said, several prominent researchers and technologists are convinced about the benefits of metformin and use it despite not being diabetic. This group includes people with their heads screwed on right. I still wouldn't recommend it, because the ability to improve health through exercise should carry more weight than the result of a single study showing a slight life extension. Single studies can be wrong, due to coincidences, errors, misunderstandings, lack of coffee at the laboratory or the wrong alignment of the stars. Personally, I need more data before using a diabetes drug with potential side effects.

But fortunately, metformin advocates are serious about their beliefs and share this conviction. They are currently arranging a more rigorous study to test out metformin in healthy people. In the upcoming TAME (Targeting Ageing with Metformin) trial, thousands of Americans will be given metformin or a placebo to test whether the drug can prolong life, by how much and at what cost. Stay tuned.

Chapter 23

What Gets Measured Gets Managed

We can survive injuries to many organs. Lose a kidney? Fine. Lose half your liver? Fine. Lose a limb? Fine. But two organs stand out as vitally important: the heart and the brain. If something bad happens to either of them, we're in deep trouble. This is visible on the list of our biggest killers. In most countries, the number one killer is cardiovascular diseases – most notably heart attacks and stroke.

Unfortunately, researchers in this field suffer from a condition that requires them to make every term as convoluted and hard to spell as possible. We want to stay healthy in old age, though, so let's give it a shot anyway.

Most cardiovascular diseases are due to something called atherosclerosis. Which is a subtype of arteriosclerosis, not to be confused with arteriolosclerosis. Yes, I know.

You can think of atherosclerosis as fatty plaque building up in the walls of your arteries, like the pipes beneath a sink slowly getting clogged. Over time (and due to the decline of ageing), this build-up can eventually cause trouble. An artery can get blocked, or a piece of fatty debris can dislodge, travel through the bloodstream and block a smaller blood vessel. In both cases the result is that downstream tissue doesn't get enough oxygen, and becomes damaged or dies. Again, this is especially bad if that tissue is in the heart (heart attack) or the brain (stroke).

We can age without much atherosclerosis, but ageing *is* a huge risk factor. Young people just don't get heart attacks. However, the initial signs of atherosclerosis can show up early in life. For instance, during the Korean War, American doctors were surprised to find that almost eighty per cent of deceased soldiers had signs of fatty plaque in the blood vessels supplying the heart. These men had an average age of twenty-two. It turns out that even *children* can have blood vessels with (very) early signs of plaque development – especially if they live with smokers.

In some genetic conditions, the process of atherosclerosis is vastly accelerated. One of them, 'familial hypercholesterolae-mia', was named to keep non-native English speakers like me awake at night. We can call it 'FH' from now on. If left untreated, people with FH have five to twenty times the normal risk of heart attacks and stroke. Half of men with untreated FH get heart attacks before turning fifty, while a third of untreated women get them before sixty. It seems whatever is happening in FH, we should seek to do the opposite.

The mutations causing FH make the liver worse at removing something called LDL cholesterol from the blood. LDL is technically a protein that transports fats around the body, but you can simply think of LDL cholesterol as 'bad cholesterol'. People with FH have much higher levels of LDL cholesterol in the blood than normal because their bodies don't remove it sufficiently. Sometimes they have so much that they develop visible yellow deposits above the eyes. Cholesterol is also a part of the fatty plaque that builds up inside arteries, so at this point we have a smoking gun.

We also know people with the opposite disposition from FH. Certain mutations in the gene PCSK9 make the liver aggressively *remove* LDL cholesterol from the blood, ensuring abnormally low levels. This condition vastly decreases the risk of heart attacks.

The case strengthens as we see the same pattern in regular people: the higher your blood LDL cholesterol levels throughout life, the higher your risk of getting heart attacks and strokes. Even within normal ranges. Lowering LDL cholesterol levels using drugs or lifestyle changes decreases the risk, and the drop is proportional to the drop in LDL cholesterol levels. Again, even within normal ranges.

Despite the overwhelming amount of evidence, some people desperately want cardiovascular diseases to be about something other than cholesterol. They have even tried constructing elaborate conspiracy theories where cholesterol is harmless and Big Bad Pharma is just out to steal our money. One reason that theory is tempting to some is that eggs are delicious, but also have a high cholesterol content. Health authorities used to vilify eggs based on the logic that eating a lot of cholesterol would increase blood levels of LDL cholesterol, causing heart attacks. However, health authorities have relaxed a bit lately. If you like eggs, you can take a deep breath, too. You see, we don't just get cholesterol from our food; our bodies can make it by themselves as well. In fact, most of the cholesterol in our bodies is not from food we've eaten, but instead has been produced by us. That means there isn't necessarily a connection between how much cholesterol you eat and how much cholesterol you have in your blood. If you eat more cholesterol, your body will simply turn its own production down.

There's some pretty intense examples of this. In one case study, doctors discovered an eighty-eight-year-old man with dementia who was eating twenty-five soft-boiled eggs a day. He had kept this habit up for years, but despite ingesting humongous amounts of cholesterol (and being old), his blood LDL cholesterol was perfectly normal. Doctors would never have suspected this man of being a real-life incarnation of the Easter Bunny if carers hadn't told them about his egg habit.

The man's secret was that his body had adapted to the unusual diet. Doctors found that he only absorbed a little of the cholesterol he ate, that he had increased cholesterol loss and that he produced little cholesterol on his own. All of this was his body's way to keep cholesterol levels in check while living on nothing but eggs.

There are similar results from studies in the 1970s and 1980s, where doctors experimented with using a diet of thirty-five eggs a day to treat patients with severe burns. Again, the patients had normal blood values for cholesterol throughout the studies, despite their gargantuan cholesterol intake.

I'm not going to recommend you try these diets, but eggs *are* delicious and also perfectly healthy. Research on more reasonable diets suggests that moderate egg consumption (one a day on average) does not increase the risk of atherosclerosis at all.

That doesn't mean we cannot influence LDL cholesterol levels using our diets, though. You might have noticed that I haven't included a ton of advice in this book in the form of 'eat this specific herb/mushroom/plant and live forever'. This is mostly because such claims are almost always false. But I'm going to make an exception here. There's actually some pretty good evidence that eating garlic (both as actual garlic and as supplements) incurs several health benefits, among them lowering LDL cholesterol levels in the blood. Researchers report the following side effects: 'Garlic odour, breath or taste was noticed in a greater proportion of participants in the active treatment group.' But despite that, I'm sure eating more garlic is a habit you can get behind.

An even better dietary trick for lowering LDL cholesterol is eating more dietary fibre. You see, we used to eat a lot more fibre than we do today. Both hunter-gatherers and medieval peasants had to actually chew their food, and one of the reasons is that they ate more foods with a high fibre content. Modern hunter-gatherers who still live like this have significantly lower LDL cholesterol levels than us, and also substantially lower risks of cardiovascular diseases.

Similarly, in modern societies, high intakes of dietary fibre are associated with living a long life. Is that just a longevity cargo cult, i.e., because rich, educated people eat more fibre?

No. Randomised controlled trials prove that dietary fibre intake lowers LDL cholesterol levels. When people add extra dietary fibre to their diets, their LDL cholesterol levels reliably fall. The mechanism is well understood, too. We can't digest dietary fibre, which means it passes through the digestive system intact. On the way, it traps something called bile acids, which we use to digest and absorb fat. Our bodies try to recycle bile acids by reabsorbing them after use, but when they get trapped by fibre, we lose them. That means the liver has to make new bile acids – and the starting material for that is cholesterol, which is recruited from the blood. This mechanism might explain why modern people tend to get high LDL cholesterol levels in the first place. By evolving on high-fibre diets, our bodies expect us to lose considerably more bile acids than we do now, and are ready to compensate with LDL cholesterol in the blood. Remove the fibre, and suddenly LDL cholesterol levels get too high.

You can get more dietary fibre in two ways. The simplest solution is to include more fibre-rich foods in your diet. Fibres from oats (for instance, in the form of oatmeal in the morning) have been particularly well-studied, but really, any fibre-rich food will do. Wholegrains, beans and fruits such as apples and pears are all excellent sources of dietary fibre. The other option is to use fibre supplements. Obviously, whole foods are preferable, but none of us is perfect. The most popular and well-documented approach is to take supplements containing psyllium. Studies usually use 5–15g a day, taken in 5g doses with one, two or three meals. (Obviously, cholesterol-lowering drugs are also an option if LDL cholesterol levels cannot be adequately controlled by diet or lifestyle.)

★ ★ ★

Another major risk factor for cardiovascular diseases is hypertension, or high blood pressure. The vast majority of people who have a heart attack or stroke have high blood pressure beforehand.

One of the important hormones involved in controlling blood pressure is called angiotensin II. When this hormone binds to its corresponding receptor, blood vessels constrict, raising blood pressure. You can think of it as squeezing on a water hose. If the same amount of water has to pass through, it will do so under higher pressure. Interestingly, there's a genetic variant in the receptor for angiotensin II that is overrepresented among centenarians. This means it might increase the likelihood of living a long life. The mechanism is straightforward: this genetic variant makes it harder for angiotensin II to activate the receptor, meaning it protects against high blood pressure.

Researchers in Italy have created mice with an extreme version of this trait by completely deactivating the angiotensin II receptor. These mice are genetically immune to high blood pressure and reap the benefits by living twenty-six per cent longer than usual. This is interesting, because you don't have to be a genetic mutant – we already have drugs that can do the same thing. When rats are treated with one of these drugs, they, too, live longer than normal. This stuff supposedly works even in the laboratory worm *C. elegans*, which is quite remarkable considering it doesn't even *have* blood vessels.

Clearly, it's a good idea to avoid high blood pressure if you want to live a long and healthy life. Unfortunately, however, blood pressure tends to increase with age. Some people say this is inevitable, but is it really?

Unknowingly, the Venezuelan government has set up a unique experiment to help us answer that question. In the Venezuelan part of the Amazon, on the border with Brazil, there are several tribes living a traditional hunter–gatherer lifestyle. That is, they hunt to get meat, gather various edible plants and have a low-tech way of life. Tribal members get plenty of exercise, but their lifestyle also provides time for relaxation and lots of social interaction.

The Venezuelan government has built a runway on the territory of one of these tribes, the Ye'kuana. In response, the tribespeople have begun trading their way to tasty processed foods when visitors arrive by air. Other tribes, such as the related Yanomami, however, still live in complete isolation on their ancestral diets.

American scientists have gone to Venezuela to study how this disparity has affected the health of the tribespeople. They found that blood pressure tends to rise with age among the runway-having Ye'kuana people, just like it does in the developed world among the rest of us. But among the isolated Yanomami, there is no age-related increase in blood pressure. When living on their ancestral diet, these people seem to age without ever getting hypertension. Scientists have found something similar among the indigenous Tsimané people of Bolivia. Here, too, blood pressure rises with age, but only when groups have access to processed food.

This suggests increasing blood pressure isn't necessarily part of getting old; it's not a 'natural' part of ageing. In fact, it might be completely avoidable. All you have to do is move to the jungle and catch your food with a spear.

Failing that, I have some advice for you that might be a little easier to implement. For instance, we've already learned about one thing that tends to increase blood pressure: cytomegalovirus (CMV) infection. It is not unlikely that other chronic viral infections do the same so vaccinations and hygiene is relevant once again.

In a pleasant surprise, it also turns out that most things you can do to lower LDL cholesterol levels work equally well for high blood pressure: eating more dietary fibre, losing weight, quitting smoking and, yes, also eating garlic.

However, there is also an additional drug that works particularly well for lowering blood pressure. Not only that, it also lowers blood sugar, increases autophagy and improves mitochondrial function.

In 1991, scientists in Cleveland began a long-term study of this drug. They recruited subjects and divided them into groups that were instructed to take increasing doses. More than fifteen years later, the scientists did a final follow-up with the subjects and published their results. They found that those taking the drug in high doses were *eighty per cent* less likely to have died compared to those not receiving the drug. It also turned out that higher dosages reliably improved the health of the subjects. The group that fared best got the highest dose, followed by those on the second-highest dose, and so it continued all the way down to those not using the drug.

. . . Okay – it wasn't actually a drug. It was exercise.

What the Cleveland scientists actually did was put people on a treadmill and measure their cardiorespiratory fitness, their 'physical shape'. During fifteen years of follow-ups, they found that those in the best shape had an eighty per cent reduced mortality risk compared to those in the worst shape – and they didn't find any plateau where exercise stopped mattering. Even at the very top, when comparing the 'elite' with those just below them, there was still a benefit to being in better shape.

★ ★ ★

It's generally not easy to study the long-term impact of exercise. You might think getting people to change their *diets* long-term is hard, but imagine getting hundreds or thousands of people to pick up a new exercise habit and stick with it for years. Due to this difficulty, most studies on exercise are correlational. In some of these studies – like the one from Cleveland above – scientists actually measure people's cardiorespiratory fitness. But in many other studies on exercise, participants are instead asked to self-report their activity levels. To everyone's surprise, it turns out most people vastly exaggerate how much they exercise.

That makes the studies less reliable – but for once, it is in a positive direction. If people don't exercise nearly as much as they claim but scientists still find benefits, that could mean exercise is even more beneficial than thought. And that we might need less exercise than expected to start reaping the benefits.

While quality long-term studies on exercise are hard to do, short-term interventions are more realistic. In these, exercise has been shown to induce all sorts of beneficial adaptations that we know are life-extending: improved mitochondrial number and function, improved insulin sensitivity, increased autophagy, improved function of the immune system, and so on.

Exercise is an example of hormesis, and as we've learned that means the benefits appear during recovery. For instance, during exercise, blood pressure, blood sugar, oxidative stress and inflammation all rise. But in the long term, exercise *decreases* resting blood pressure, *improves* blood sugar levels and *decreases* inflammation and oxidative stress. We adapt to the stress of exercise by becoming more resilient. However, as exercise works by hormesis, it is also clear that there must be a ceiling somewhere: some tipping point where the stress factor becomes too big. The question is whether that ceiling for exercise is anything normal people like you and I should worry about. In other words, whether you bump into it hobby-jogging a few times a week, or whether it is only applicable if you try out Race Across America or Marathon des Sables.

According to the study from Cleveland, we have nothing to worry about. Even the most active participants fared well, and we can safely live by the rule that more exercise is better. But obviously, this is one of those things where you have to listen to your body. Remember that exercise is healthy because of all the things that happen while you recover.

The traditional way to exercise is so-called 'steady-state' exercise. Here, you get your pulse up, exert yourself at a moderate level and remain active for long periods of time. Examples could be running, cycling, swimming or even hiking. These habits are great, but they're vulnerable to the number one anti-exercise excuse: 'I don't have the time.' If someone claims they have never used this one, they're probably lying. A potential solution is interval training, also known as 'high-intensity interval training' (HIIT). In HIIT, short periods of intense activity are alternated with rest periods. For instance, twenty seconds of sprinting, twenty seconds of rest, twenty seconds of sprinting, and so on, continued for five to fifteen minutes. The aim is to reach higher levels of exertion than during steady-state exercise. This can be beneficial, as hormesis often works best with high-intensity acute stressors. Proponents believe HIIT is as beneficial as steady-state exercise, and studies tend to back this up. Among other things, a large meta-analysis has shown that interval training reduces inflammation and oxidative stress more than steady-state training – and at the same time, it also increases insulin sensitivity more. Another study has shown that interval training leads to approximately twenty-five per cent more weight loss than moderate steady-state training.

The optimal fitness regimen might include both steady-state and interval training. For instance, a runner could go jogging as usual and also sometimes do sprint intervals. However, it is important to not let the perfect get in the way of the good. Studies show that all activity is better than none, and the very best is exercising as a regular habit. That's a lot easier if you pick something you like.

There's a kind of mouse that would best be described as a 'muscle mouse'. These mice have twice as much muscle mass as regular mice and also carry less body fat. They're everything human bodybuilders dream about, without having to live at the gym or eat excessive amounts of boiled chicken. These muscle mice are extra muscular because they have defects in a gene called myostatin. Myostatin normally inhibits muscle growth, so if it stops working, muscles will grow larger. Interestingly, we also know other animals with myostatin defects: cows, dogs, sheep and, yes, also humans. In 2004, for instance, a boy was born in Germany with mutations in both his myostatin genes. Doctors described him as 'extremely muscular', even as a new-born. Unsurprisingly, his mother was an athlete.

Myostatin is particularly interesting to us because the muscle mice are not just extremely muscular – they also live longer than regular mice. Myostatin works similarly in most mammals, so perhaps we should be lowering our myostatin levels as well. I'm sure someone will eventually figure out a way to do this medically without side effects, and so join the Silicon Valley guys at the top of the *Forbes* list. For now, though, the best option is the old-fashioned one: lifting weights. One of the ways weightlifting makes muscles increase in size over time is exactly by lowering our myostatin levels.

As we age, we tend to lose muscle mass. An eighty-year-old person has lost an average of fifty per cent of their muscle fibres. This is the reason people get weaker with age – and it also decreases resilience in the face of disease. People with low muscle mass or grip strength tend to die younger, but weightlifting can help in two ways. First, if we start from a larger muscle mass, it takes a longer time to decline down to a point where low muscle mass becomes a problem. Second, weightlifting can also counteract the actual muscle loss by way of hormesis. The weight-bearing stress forces the body to invest in muscle upkeep and strengthening. Similarly, weightlifting also counteracts age-related loss of bone density. Many older people, especially older women, have problems with osteoporosis – hollowed-out and fragile bones. Again, this can be counteracted by taxing bones through weightlifting. So the conclusion is that while aerobic exercise is the most important exercise for longevity it is highly beneficial to also include weightlifting. The absolute ideal programme, if you can bear it, would probably include both steady-state training, interval training and weightlifting.

Chapter 24

Mind Over Matter

Imagine that we're a pair of doctors who are visited by our friend John. John complains about a headache, and we tell him that, sure, we have a pill for that. But instead of giving John a pain reliever, we deceive him. We tell him he's getting a drug, but it's actually just a sugar pill. John thanks us and swallows the pill with a glass of water.

Now, the sugar pill should have no medical effect whatsoever. But soon, John starts lightening up and he thanks us for curing his headache. Is John a liar?

No. What John is experiencing is a classic effect in medicine called the placebo effect. This is a phenomenon where one's expectations end up having an actual medical impact. In other words, it's when a drug works not because of some high-tech molecular reason, but because patients *think* it works. There's a lot to suggest the placebo effect is an important part of most medical treatment, especially when there's a mental component involved. As a result, the placebo effect can be enhanced in accordance with the strength of a patient's belief. It works even better if the patient thinks the drug is brand new, if it is expensive, if the pill is really big or – for some reason – if it is red.

Treating headaches with sugar pills is interesting, but there are also far more bizarre examples out there – for instance, the use of placebo *surgery*. In one study, a group of researchers were treating patients with osteoarthritis of the knee. This is a painful condition that is hard to treat, but which can sometimes be alleviated using surgery. Doctors put osteoarthritis patients under anaesthesia and then made surgical incisions in their knees. However, only a few of the patients had the actual surgery. The rest were simply sewn back together with no intervention other than the original cut. The doctors didn't tell the patients, who assumed that they'd had an actual surgery. And incredibly, during the following months, the placebo version of the surgery worked just as well as the real surgery, with the two patient groups reporting an equal decrease in pain.

There are even studies where doctors are completely honest about their use of placebos. They tell patients, 'This is just a placebo treatment, we're not actually doing anything. However, previous studies show that placebo treatments work.' And then the treatment does end up working. In one study, for example, doctors gave sugar pills to patients with irritable bowel syndrome and were open about what they were doing. Nevertheless, patients' symptoms improved.

I guess the good news is that the advice in this book will help you live longer providing I've managed to convince you I'm right. Okay, living for a long time might require a little more than 'believe, achieve', but studies do show that people who *feel* younger than their actual age tend to live longer. Similarly, we also know optimistic people tend to live longer.

The placebo effect illustrates that our mental state is in the driver's seat of the body. It can even affect how we react to food. In a fascinating study, scientists made participants drink a sugary drink. Some were told the drink was a high-sugar beverage, while others were told the opposite. Then, even though both groups drank identical drinks, *their bodies reacted differently.* People thinking they were drinking a high-sugar drink had higher blood sugar spikes than those who thought they were drinking a low-sugar drink.

And this is the flipside of the placebo coin. The placebo effect also has an evil twin: the nocebo effect. Here, *negative* expectations become self-fulfilling. A good example is a study where researchers purported to measure people's genetic potential for getting in good physical shape. Scientists told some of the research participants that they were predisposed to being in bad shape, even if it was a complete lie. Subsequently, those people performed worse on physical tests than people told the opposite.

★ ★ ★

Owning a dog is associated with living longer. The same is true of having close family relationships and friendships. In one study, researchers reviewed autobiographies and compared how often words for social roles appeared in the books; for instance, words like father, mother, siblings and neighbour. The authors who used these kinds of words the most lived over six years longer than those who used them the least.

We see this connection because all the tips and tricks in this book are not enough. Eating a healthy diet, exercising, and experimenting with your lifestyle will get you a long way. But it won't take you to the finish line.

The final ingredient we're missing is our social relationships. We now know how important our psychological state is to our physical health. And as human beings, one of our deepest psychological needs is belonging somewhere. For this rea-son, loneliness is actually among the factors most strongly associated with an early death – more so than being over-weight, for instance. The need for close social ties is so ancient that we share it with our distant relatives. Even among baboons, the individuals who have stronger social ties live longer than individuals with weak and unstable social ties.

In addition to the happiness and comfort being with other people gives us, we also derive great meaning and a sense of duty from our social relationships. Field studies on longevity consistently find that long-lived people have powerful senses of meaning and purpose, and are exceptionally engaged in the world at any age. Instead of dividing life into 'work' and 'pension', they continue to take on tasks and responsibilities throughout their lives, even at the point where this has dwindled down to 'cook for my grandchildren every Sunday' or simply 'sweep the stairs every day'. A curious example is that death rates rose right after the turn of the millennium. It's as if people were kept alive by their goal of experiencing the new millennium, and didn't give in until they'd got there.

Epilogue

Our search for the secrets of a long and healthy life has taken us around the world, from the Greenland Sea to Easter Island and the African tunnel kingdoms of the naked mole-rat. Along the way, we have met old-school adventurers, self-experimentalists and, of course, some of the best scientists in the world. Whoever you are and wherever you're reading this book, I hope you enjoyed the ride.

Research on ageing is still in its infancy, but as we've learned, we have made many important strides already. In the years to come, the snowball will keep rolling. The question of why we age and, more importantly, what to do about it, is one of the oldest questions there is. Older even than civilisation itself. As this book proves, we're as interested as ever.

The usual pessimists might decry the ambition to live a longer life, but the fight against ageing is a noble one. There is so much in this world that drives us apart. We've learned the hard way that one of the best ways to unite people is through a common enemy. For once, we have the chance to turn this into a good thing. Everyone is going to age, no matter their ethnicity, nationality, sex, income level or education. We're all in it together, and that also means any progress made is applicable to all of us.

Provided we can continue our progress in medical science, there's no doubt we will eventually defeat ageing. The only question is when. I hope someone finds this book in fifty years' time, smiles at its simplicity and is grateful for the many discoveries that have come after. But whether the fight against ageing will take 50, 500 or 5,000 years, no one knows. At one point, a generation will be born that is the last generation to be ravaged by ageing. We could hope that it would be us, but alas we might not be that lucky.

– Nicklas Brendborg, Copenhagen (2022)

Acknowledgements

I want to thank my wonderful editor Izzy Everington and the rest of the team at Hodder Studio for their hard work making this book. With their help it has exceeded my wildest expectations. Thanks also to Elizabeth deNoma, who helped translate the original Danish book; Tara O'Sullivan, who helped spice up my English during editing; Lydia Blagden for the beautiful design of the cover; and Purvi Gadia for her diligence in guiding this book through its final stages.

I also want to thank my agent, Paul Sebes, Rik Kleuver, and the rest of the team at Sebes & Bisseling Literary Agency. Due to their brilliance, this book has truly gone global. At the time of writing it has been translated into twenty-two languages all over the world with no signs of slowing down. Getting a call from Paul and Rik is always exciting, but I'm particularly grateful for their instrumental part in making this translation possible – the translation into English, both the world language and the language of science.

I must also mention my lovely Danish publishers Louise Vind and Marianne Kiertzner at Forlaget Grønningen 1. Believe it or not, this book was rejected by every single major publisher in my home country at first. In fact, it took me longer to get it published than it took to actually write it. Fortunately, I eventually met Louise and Marianne who didn't take long to make up their minds. The rest is history – our first print sold out on the day of the launch and *Jellyfish Age Backwards* became the number one bestselling nonfiction book of the year.

Finally, I want to thank all my loved ones and dedicate this book to them. The reason I want to stick around for a long time is to make many more memories with you guys.

Bibliography

Introduction: The Fountain of Youth

Conese, M., Carbone, A., Beccia, E., Angiolillo. A. 'The Fountain of Youth: A tale of parabiosis, stem cells, and rejuvenation', *Open Medicine*, vol. 12, 2017, pp. 376–383.

Grundhauser, E. 'The True Story of Dr. Voronoff's Plan to Use Monkey Testicles to Make Us Immortal', atlasobscura.com, 13 October 2015.

Chapter 1: The Record Book of Longevity

Nielsen, J. et al. 'Eye lens radiocarbon reveals centuries of longevity in the Greenland shark (*Somniosus microcephalus*)', *Science*, vol. 353, no. 6300, 2016, pp. 702–704.

Keane, M. et al. 'Insights into the evolution of longevity from the bowhead whale genome', *Cell Reports*, vol. 10, no. 1, 2015, pp. 112–122.

Bailey, D.K. '*Pinus Longaeva*', *The Gymnosperm Database*, www.conifers.org/pi/Pinus_longaeva.php.

Rogers, P., McAvoy, D. 'Mule deer impede Pando's recovery: Implications for aspen resilience from a single-genotype forest', *PLOS ONE*, vol. 13, no. 10, 2017.

Robb, J., Turbott, E. '*Tu'i Malila*, "Cook's Tortoise"', *Records of the Auckland Institute and Museum*, vol. 8, 17 December 1971, pp. 229–233.

Morbey, Y., Brassil, C., Hendry, A. 'Rapid Senescence in Pacific Salmon', *The American Naturalist*, vol. 166, no. 5, 2005, pp. 556–568.

Wang, Z., Ragsdale, C. 'Multiple optic gland signaling pathways implicated in octopus maternal behaviors and death', *Journal of Experimental Biology*, vol. 221, no. 19, 2018.

Bradley, A., McDonald, I., Lee, A. 'Stress and mortality in a small marsupial (*Antechinus stuartii*, Macleay)', *General and Comparative Endocrinology*, vol. 40, no. 2, 1980, pp. 188–200.

White, J., Lloyd, M. '17-Year Cicadas Emerging After 18 Years: A New Brood?' *Evolution*, vol. 33, no. 4, 1979, pp. 1193–1199.

Sweeney, B., Vannote, R. 'Population Synchrony in Mayflies: A Predator Satiation Hypothesis', *Evolution*, vol. 36, no. 4, 1982, pp. 810–821.

'Century plant', *Encyclopaedia Britannica*, www.britannica.com/plant/century-plant-Agave-genus, 2020.

Bavestrello, G., Sommer, C., Sarà, M. 'Bi-directional conversion in *Turritopsis nutricula* (Hydrozoa)', *Scientia Marina*, vol. 56, no. 2–3, 1992, pp. 137–140.

Carla', E., Pagliara, P., Piraino, S., Boero, F., Dini, L. 'Morphological and ultrastructural analysis of *Turritopsis nutricula* during life cycle reversal', *Tissue and Cell*, vol. 35, no. 3, 2003, pp. 213–222.

Kubota, S. 'Repeating rejuvenation in *Turritopsis*, an immortal hydrozoan (Cnidaria, Hydrozoa)', *Biogeography*, vol. 13, 2011, pp. 101–103.

Bowen, I., Ryder, T., Dark, C. 'The effects of starvation on the planarian worm *Polycelis tenuis iijima*', *Cell and Tissue Research*, vol. 169, no. 2, 1976, pp. 193–209.

Bidle, K., Lee, S., Marchant, D., Falkowski, P. 'Fossil genes and microbes in the oldest ice on Earth', *Proceedings of the National Academy of Sciences of the United States of America*, vol. 104, no. 33, 2007, pp. 13455–13460.

Austad, S. 'Retarded senescence in an insular population of Virginia opossums (*Didelphis virginiana*)', *Journal of Zoology*, vol. 229, no. 4, 1993, pp. 695–708.

Austad, S., Fischer, K. 'Mammalian Aging, Metabolism, and Ecology: Evidence From the Bats and Marsupials', *Journal of Gerontology*, vol. 46, no. 2, 1991, pp. B47–B53.

Wodinsky, J. 'Hormonal inhibition of feeding and death in Octopus: Control by optic gland secretion', *Science*, vol. 198, no. 4320, 1977, pp. 948–951.

Lewis, K., Buffenstein, R. 'The Naked Mole-Rat: A Resilient Rodent Model of Aging, Longevity, and Healthspan', *Handbook of the Biology of Aging: Eighth Edition*, Elsevier Inc., 2015, pp. 179–204.

Buffenstein, R. 'Naked mole-rat (*Heterocephalus glaber*) longevity, ageing, and life history', *An Age: The Animal and Longevity Database*, https://genomics.senescence.info.

Sahm, A. et al. 'Long-lived rodents reveal signatures of positive selection in genes associated with lifespan', *P Lo S Genetics*, vol. 14, no. 3, 2018.

Chapter 2: Sun, Palm Trees and Eternal Life

Buettner, D. *The Blue Zones: 9 lessons for living longer from the people who've lived the longest*, National Geographic Books, 2008.

Poulain, M., Herm, A., Pes, G. 'The Blue Zones: areas of exceptional longevity around the world', *Vienna Yearbook of Population Research*, vol. 11, 2013, pp. 87–108.

Rosero-Bixby, L., Dow, W., Rehkopf, D. 'The Nicoya region of Costa Rica: A high longevity Island for elderly males', *Vienna Yearbook of Population Research*, vol. 11, no. 1, 2013, pp. 109–136.

Hokama, T., Binns, C. 'Declining longevity advantage and low birthweight in Okinawa', *Asia-Pacific Journal of Public Health*, vol. 20, October 2008, suppl: 95–101.

Newman, S. J. 'Supercentenarians and the oldest-old are concentrated into regions with no birth certificates and short lifespans', *bioRxiv*, 704080, May 2020, doi: https://doi.org/10.1101/704080.

'2019 Human Development Report', United Nations Development Program, 2019.

'Life expectancy at birth, total (years)', The World Bank, 2020, https://data.worldbank.org/indicator/SP.DYN.LE00.IN.

'More than 230,000 Japanese centenarians "missing"', *BBC*, September 2010.

Chapter 3: Genes Are Overrated

Segal, N. 'Twins: A window into human nature', TEDx, Manhattan Beach, 2017, www.ted.com/talks/nancy_segal_twins_a_window_into_human_nature.

Herskind, A., McGue, M., Holm, N., Sørensen, T., Harvald, B., Vaupel, J. 'The heritability of human longevity: A population-based study of 2872 Danish twin pairs born 1870–1900', *Human Genetics*, vol. 97, no. 3, 1996, pp. 319–323.

Mitchell, B., Hsueh, W., King, T., Pollin, T., Sorkin, J., Agarwala, R., Schäffer, A., Shuldiner, A. 'Heritability of life span in the Old Order Amish', *American Journal of Medical Genetics*, vol. 102, no. 4, 2001, pp. 346–352.

Kerber, R., O'Brien, E., Smith, K., Cawthon, R. 'Familial excess longevity in Utah genealogies', *Journals of Gerontology, Series A: Biological Sciences and Medical Sciences*, vol. 56, no. 3, 2001, pp. B130–B139.

Ljungquist, B., Berg, S., Lanke, J., McClearn, G., Pedersen, N. 'The effect of genetic factors for longevity: A comparison of identical and fraternal twins in the Swedish Twin Registry', *Journals of Gerontology, Series A: Biological Sciences and Medical Sciences*, vol. 53, no. 6, 1998, pp. M441–M446.

Graham Ruby, J. et al. 'Estimates of the heritability of human longevity are substantially inflated due to assortative mating', *Genetics*, vol. 210, no. 3, 2018, pp. 1109–1124.

Melzer, D., Pilling, L.C., Ferrucci, L. 'The genetics of human ageing', *Nature Reviews Genetics*, vol. 21, 2020, pp. 88–101.

Timmers, P. et al. 'Genomics of 1 million parent lifespans implicates novel pathways and common diseases and distinguishes survival chances', *eLife*, vol. 8, 2019.

Lio, D., Pes, G., Carru, C., Listì, F., Ferlazzo, V., Candore, G., Colonna-Romano, G., Ferrucci, L., Deiana, L., Baggio, G., Franceschi,

C., Caruso, C. 'Association between the HLA-DR alleles and longevity: A study in Sardinian population', *Experimental Gerontology*, vol. 38, no. 3, 2003, pp. 313–318.

Sun, X., Chen, W., Wang, Y. 'DAF-16/FOXO transcription factor in aging and longevity', *Frontiers in Pharmacology*, vol. 8, 2017.

Raygani, A., Zahrai, M., Raygani, A., Doosti, M., Javadi, E., Rezaei, M., Pourmotabbed, T. 'Association between apolipoprotein E polymorphism and Alzheimer disease in Tehran, Iran', *Neuroscience Letters*, vol. 375, no. 1, 2005, pp. 1–6.

Liu, S., Liu, J., Weng, R., Gu, X., Zhong, Z. 'Apolipoprotein E gene polymorphism and the risk of cardiovascular disease and type 2 diabetes', *BMC Cardiovascular Disorders*, vol. 19, no. 1, 2019, p. 213.

Zook, N., Yoder, S. 'Twelve Largest Amish Settlements, 2017', Center for Anabaptist and Pietist Studies, Elizabethtown College, 2017, https://groups.etown.edu/amishstudies/statistics/largest-settlements.

Khan, S, Shah, S. et al. 'A null mutation in SERPINE1 protects against biological aging in humans', *Science Advances*, vol. 3, no. 11, 2017.

Chapter 4: The Disadvantages of Immortality

Shklovskii, B.I. 'A simple derivation of the Gompertz law for human mortality', *Theory in Biosciences*, vol. 123, 2005, pp. 431–433.

Christensen, K., McGue, M., Peterson, I., Jeune, B., Vaupel, J.W. 'Exceptional longevity does not result in excessive levels of disability', *Proceedings of the National Academy of Sciences of the United States of America*, vol. 105, no. 36, 2008, pp. 13274–13279. doi:10.1073/pnas.0804931105.

Heron, M. 'Deaths: Leading Causes for 2019', *National Vital Statistics Report*, National Center for Health Statistics, vol. 70, no. 9, 2021. doi: https://dx.doi. org/10.15620/cdc:10702.

Arias, E., Heron, M., Tejada-Vera, B. *National Vital Statistics Reports*, vol. 61, no. 9, 31 May 2013.

Arancio, W., Pizzolanti, G., Genovese, S., Pitrone, M., Giordano, C. 'Epigenetic Involvement in Hutchinson-Gilford Progeria Syndrome: A Mini-Review', *Gerontology*, vol. 60, no. 3, 2014, pp. 197–203.

Medawar, P. *An Unsolved Problem of Biology*, H.K. Lewis, 1952.

Fabian, D. 'The evolution of aging', *Nature Education Knowledge*, vol. 3, 2011, pp. 1–10.

Loison, A. et al. 'Age specific survival in five populations of ungulates: evidence of senescence', *Ecology*, vol. 80, no. 8, 1999, pp. 2539–2554.

Williams, G. 'Pleiotropy, Natural Selection, and the Evolution of Senescence', *Evolution*, vol. 11, no. 4, 1957, pp. 398–411.

Friedman, D., Johnson, T. 'A mutation in the age-1 gene in Caenorhabditis elegans lengthens life and reduces hermaphrodite fertility', *Genetics*, vol. 118, no. 1, 1988.

Chapter 5: What Doesn't Kill You...

Denham, H. 'Aging: A Theory Based on Free Radical and Radiation Chemistry', *Journal of Gerontology*, vol. 11(3): pp. 298–300, 1956. https://doi.org/10.1093/geronj/11.3.298

Bjelakovic, G., Nikolova, D., Gluud, L.L., Simonetti, R.G., Gluud, C. 'Mortality in randomized trials of antioxidant supplements for primary and secondary prevention: systematic review and meta-analysis', *JAMA*, 297(8):842–57, 2007. doi: 10.1001/jama.297.8.842.

Yang, W., Hekimi, S. 'A Mitochondrial Superoxide Signal Triggers Increased Longevity in *Caenorhabditis elegans*', *PLOS Biology*, vol. 8, no. 12, 2010.

Hwang, S., Guo, H. et al. 'Cancer risks in a population with prolonged low dose-rate γ-radiation exposure in radio-contaminated buildings, 1983–2002', *International Journal of Radiation Biology*, vol. 82, no. 12, 2006, pp. 849–858.

Sponsler, R., Cameron, J. 'Nuclear shipyard worker study (1980-1988): a large cohort exposed to low-dose-rate gamma radiation', *International Journal of Low Radiation*, vol. 1, no. 4, 2005, pp. 463–478.

David, E., Wolfson, M., Fraifeld, V. 'Background radiation impacts human longevity and cancer mortality: Reconsidering the linear no-threshold paradigm', *Biogerontology*, vol. 22, no. 2, 2021, pp. 189–195.

Berrington, A., Darby, S., Weiss, H., Doll, R. '100 years of observation on British radiologists: Mortality from cancer and other causes 1897–1997', *British Journal of Radiology*, vol. 74, no. 882, 2001, pp. 507–519.

McDonald, J. *et al.* 'Ionizing radiation activates the Nrf2 antioxidant response', *Cancer Research*, vol. 70, no. 21, 2010, pp. 8886–8895.

Nabavi, S.F., Barber, A.J., et al. 'Nrf2 as molecular target for polyphenols: A novel therapeutic strategy in diabetic retinopathy', *Critical Reviews in Clinical Laboratory Sciences*, vol. 53(5), 2016. https://doi.org/10.3109/10408363.2015.1129530.

Chaurasiya, R., Sakhare, P., Bhaskar, N., Hebbar, H. 'Efficacy of reverse micellar extracted fruit bromelain in meat tenderization', *Journal of Food Science and Technology*, vol. 52, no. 6, 2015, pp. 3870–3880.

Montgomery, M., Hulbert, A., Buttemer, W. 'Does the oxidative stress theory of aging explain longevity differences in birds? I. Mitochondrial ROS production', *Experimental Gerontology*, vol. 47, no. 3, 2012, pp. 203–210.

Lewis, K., Andziak, B., Yang, T., Buffenstein, R. 'The naked mole-rat response to oxidative stress: Just deal with it', *Antioxidants and Redox Signaling*, vol. 19, no. 12, 2013, pp. 1388–1399.

Burtscher, M. 'Lower mortality rates in those living at moderate altitude', *Aging*, vol. 8, no. 100, 2016, pp. 2603–2604.

Faeh, D., Gutzwiller, F., Bopp, M. 'Lower mortality from coronary heart disease and stroke at higher altitudes in Switzerland', *Circulation*, vol. 120, no. 6, 2009, pp. 495–501.

Baibas, N., Trichopoulou, A., Voridis, E., Trichopoulos, D. 'Residence in mountainous compared with lowland areas in relation to total and coronary mortality. A study in rural Greece', *Journal of Epidemiology and Community Health*, vol. 59, no. 4, 2005, pp. 274–278.

Thielke, S., Slatore, C., Banks, W. 'Association between Alzheimer, dementia, mortality rate and altitude in California counties',
JAMA Psychiatry, vol. 72, no. 12, 2015, pp. 1253–1254.

Laukkanen, J., Laukkanen, T., Kunutsor, S. 'Cardiovascular and Other Health Benefits of Sauna Bathing: A Review of the Evidence',
Mayo Clinic Proceedings, vol. 93, no. 8, 2018, pp. 1111–1121.

Darcy, J., Tseng, Y. 'ComBATing aging – does increased brown
adipose tissue activity confer longevity?', *GeroScience*, vol. 41,
no. 3, 2019, pp. 285–296.

Schmeisser, S., Schmeisser, K. et al. 'Mitochondrial hormesis links
low-dose arsenite exposure to lifespan extension', *Aging Cell*,
vol. 12, no. 3, 2013, pp. 508–517.

Oelrichs, P., MacLeod, J., Seawright, A., Ng, J. 'Isolation and char-
acterisation of urushiol components from the Australian native
cashew (*Semecarpus australiensis*)', *Natural Toxins*, vol. 5, no. 3,
1998, pp. 96–98.

Jonak, C., Klosner, G., Trautinger, F. 'Significance of heat shock proteins in the skin upon UV exposure', *Frontiers in Bioscience*, vol.
14 no. 12, 2009, pp. 4758–4768.

Chapter 6: Does Size Matter?

Laron, Z., Lilos, P., Klinger, B. 'Growth curves for Laron syndrome',
Archives of Disease in Childhood, vol. 68, no. 6, 1993, pp. 768–770.

Guevara-Aguirre, J. et al. 'Growth hormone receptor deficiency is
associated with a major reduction in pro-aging signaling, cancer,
and diabetes in humans', *Science Translational Medicine*, vol. 3,
no. 70, 2011.

Bartke, A,, Brown-Borg, H. 'Life Extension in the Dwarf Mouse',
Current Topics in Developmental Biology, vol. 63, 2004, pp. 189–225.

Salaris, L., Poulain, M., Samaras, T. 'Height and survival at older ages
among men born in an inland village in Sardinia (Italy), 1866-2006',
Biodemography and Social Biology, vol. 58, no. 1, 2012, pp. 1–13.

Samaras, T., Elrick, H., Storms, L. 'Is height related to longevity?',
Life Sciences, vol. 72, no. 16, 2003, pp. 1781–1802.

Kurosu, H. et al. 'Physiology: Suppression of aging in mice by the hormone Klotho', *Science*, vol. 309, no. 5742, 2005, pp. 1829–1833.

Vitale, G. et al. 'Low circulating IGF-I bioactivity is associated with human longevity: Findings in centenarians' offspring', *Aging*, vol. 4, no. 9, 2012, pp. 580–589.

Zarse, K. et al. 'Impaired insulin/IGF1 signaling extends life span by promoting mitochondrial L-proline catabolism to induce a transient ROS signal', *Cell Metabolism*, vol. 15, no. 4, 2012, pp. 451–465.

Zoledziewska, M. et al. 'Height-reducing variants and selection for short stature in Sardinia', *Nature Genetics*, vol. 47, no. 11, 2015, pp. 1352–1356.

Wolkow, C., Kimura, K., Lee, M., Ruvkun, G. 'Regulation of *C. elegans* life span by insulin-like signaling in the nervous system', *Science*, vol. 290, no. 5489, 2000, pp. 147–150.

Chapter 7: The Secrets of Easter Island

Halford, B. 'Rapamycin's secrets unearthed', *C&EN Global Enterprise*, vol. 94, no. 29, 2016, pp. 26–30.

Dominick, G. et al. 'Regulation of mTOR Activity in Snell Dwarf and GH Receptor Gene-Disrupted Mice', *Endocrinology*, vol. 156, no. 2, 2015, pp. 565–75.

Sharp, Z., Bartke, A. 'Evidence for Down-Regulation of Phosphoinositide 3-Kinase/Akt/Mammalian Target of Rapamycin (PI3K/Akt/mTOR)-Dependent Translation Regulatory Signaling Pathways in Ames Dwarf Mice', *The Journals of Gerontology, Series A: Biological Sciences and Medical Sciences*, vol. 60, no. 3, 2005, pp. 293–300.

Bitto, A. et al. 'Transient rapamycin treatment can increase lifespan and healthspan in middle-aged mice', *Elife*, vol. 5, 2016.

Zhang, Y. et al. 'Rapamycin Extends Life and Health in C57BL/6 Mice', *The Journals of Gerontology, Series A: Biological Sciences and Medical Sciences*, vol. 69A, no. 2, 2014.

Mannick, J. et al. 'TORC1 inhibition enhances immune function and reduces infections in the elderly', *Science Translational Medicine*, vol. 10, no. 449, 2018, p. 1564.

Arriola Apelo, S., Lamming, D. 'Rapamycin: An InhibiTOR of aging emerges from the soil of Easter Island', *The Journals of Gerontology, Series A: Biological Sciences and Medical Sciences*, vol. 71, no. 7, 2016, pp. 841–849.

Leidal, A., Levine, B., Debnath, J. 'Autophagy and the cell biology of age-related disease', *Nature Cell Biology*, vol. 20, 2018, pp. 1338–1348.

Dai, D. et al. 'Altered proteome turnover and remodeling by short-term caloric restriction or rapamycin rejuvenate the aging heart', *Aging Cell*, vol. 13, no. 3, 2014, pp. 529–539.

Bitto, A. et al. 'Transient rapamycin treatment can increase lifespan and healthspan in middle-aged mice', *eLife*, vol. 5, 2016.

Chapter 8: The One to Unite Them All

Mujahid N. et al. 'A UV-Independent Topical Small-Molecule Approach for Melanin Production in Human Skin', *CellReports*, vol. 19, 2017, pp. 2177–2184.

'The Nobel Prize in Physiology or Medicine 2016', NobelPrize.org, 2020.

Kumsta, C., Chang, J., Schmalz, J., Hansen, M. 'Hormetic heat stress and HSF-1 induce autophagy to improve survival and proteostasis in *C. Elegans*', *Nature Communications*, vol. 8, no. 1, 2017, pp. 1–12.

Rodriguez, K. et al. 'Walking the Oxidative Stress Tightrope: A Perspective from the Naked Mole-Rat, the Longest-Living Rodent', *Current Pharmaceutical Design*, vol. 17, no. 22, 2011, pp. 2290–2307.

Kacprzyk, J., Locatelli, A. et al. 'Evolution of mammalian longevity: age-related increase in autophagy in bats compared to other mammals', *Aging*, vol. 13, no. 6, 2021, pp. 7998–8025.

Pugin, B. et al. 'A wide diversity of bacteria from the human gut produces and degrades biogenic amines', *Microbial Ecology in Health and Disease*, vol. 28, no. 1, 2017.

Eisenberg, T. et al. 'Cardioprotection and lifespan extension by the natural polyamine spermidine', *Nature Medicine*, vol. 22, no. 12, 2016, pp. 1428–1438.

Kiechl, S. et al. 'Higher spermidine intake is linked to lower mortality: A prospective population-based study', *American Journal of Clinical Nutrition*, vol. 108, no. 2, 2018, pp. 371–380.

Nishimura, K., Shiina, R., Kashiwagi, K., Igarashi, K. 'Decrease in Polyamines with Aging and Their Ingestion from Food and Drink', *The Journal of Biochemistry*, vol. 139, no. 1, 2006, pp. 81–90.

Chapter 9: Infamous High School Biology

Crane, J., Devries, M., Safdar, A., Hamadeh, M., Tarnopolsky, M. 'The effect of aging on human skeletal muscle mitochondrial and intramyocellular lipid ultrastructure', *Journals of Gerontology, Series A: Biological Sciences and Medical Sciences*, vol. 65, no. 2, 2010, pp. 119–128.

Conley, K., Jubrias, S., Esselman, P. 'Oxidative capacity and ageing in human muscle', *Journal of Physiology*, vol. 526, no. 1, 2000, pp. 203–210.

Picca, A. et al. 'Update on mitochondria and muscle aging: All wrong roads lead to sarcopenia', *Biological Chemistry*, vol. 399, no. 5, 2018, pp. 421–436.

Sun, N. et al. 'Measuring In Vivo Mitophagy,' *Molecular Cell*, vol. 60, no. 4, 2015, pp. 685–696.

Oliveira, A., Hood, D. 'Exercise is mitochondrial medicine for muscle', *Sports Medicine and Health Science*, vol. 1, no. 1, 2019, pp. 11–18.

Van Remmen, H. et al. 'Life-long reduction in MnSOD activity results in increased DNA damage and higher incidence of cancer but does not accelerate aging', *Physiological Genomics*, vol. 16, no. 1, 2004, pp. 29–37.

Zhang, Y. et al. 'Mice deficient in both Mn superoxide dismutase and glutathione peroxidase-1 have increased oxidative damage and a greater incidence of pathology but no reduction in longevity,' *Journals of Gerontology, Series A: Biological Sciences and Medical Sciences*, vol. 64, no. 12, 2009, pp. 1212–1220.

Andreux, P.A. et al. 'The mitophagy activator urolithin A is safe and induces a molecular signature of improved mitochondrial and cellular health in humans', *Nature Metabolism*, vol. 1, no. 6, 2019, pp. 595–603.

Chapter 10: Adventures in Immortality

M. Funk, 'Liz Parrish Wants to Live Forever', outsideonline.com, 18 July 2018.

Okuda, K., Bardeguez, A. et al. 'Telomere Length in the Newborn', *Pediatric Research*, vol. 52. no. 3, 2002, pp. 377–381.

Armanios, M., Blackburn, E. 'The telomere syndromes', *Nature Reviews Genetics*, vol. 13, no. 10, 2012, pp. 693–704.

Arai, Y. et al. 'Inflammation, But Not Telomere Length, Predicts Successful Ageing at Extreme Old Age: A Longitudinal Study of Semi-supercentenarians', *eBio Medicine*, vol. 2, no. 10, 2015, pp. 1549–1558.

Hayflick, L., Moorhead, P. 'The serial cultivation of human diploid cell strains', *Experimental Cell Research*, vol. 25, no. 3, 1961, pp. 585–621.

'The Nobel Prize in Physiology or Medicine 2009', NobelPrize.org, 2020.

Cawthon, R., Smith, K., O'Brien, E., Sivatchenko, A., Kerber, R. 'Association between telomere length in blood and mortality in people aged 60 years or older', *Lancet*, vol. 361, no. 9355, 2003, pp. 393–395.

Shay, J., Bacchetti, S. 'A survey of telomerase activity in human cancer', *European Journal of Cancer Part A*, vol. 33, no. 5, 1997, pp. 787–791.

Rode, L., Nordestgaard, B., Bojesen, S. 'Long telomeres and cancer risk among 95,568 individuals from the general population', *International Journal of Epidemiology*, vol. 45, no. 5, 2016.

Pellatt, A. et al. 'Telomere length, telomere-related genes, and breast cancer risk: The breast cancer health disparities study', *Genes, Chromosomes and Cancer*, vol. 52, no. 7, 2013.

Nan, H., Du, M. et al. 'Shorter telomeres associate with a reduced risk of melanoma development', *Cancer Research*, vol. 71, no. 21, pp. 6758–6763.

Kuo, C., Pilling, L., Kuchel, G., Ferrucci, L., Melzer, D. 'Telomere length and aging-related outcomes in humans: A Mendelian randomization study in 261,000 older participants', *Aging Cell*, vol. 18, no. 6, 2019.

Garrett-Bakelman, F. et al. 'The NASA twins study: A multidimensional analysis of a year-long human spaceflight', *Science*, vol. 364, no. 6436, 2019.

Chapter 11: Zombie Cells and How to Get Rid of Them

'The Nobel Prize in Physiology or Medicine 2016', NobelPrize.org, 2020.

Takahashi, K., Yamanaka, S. 'Induction of Pluripotent Stem Cells from Mouse Embryonic and Adult Fibroblast Cultures by Defined Factors', *Cell*, vol. 126, no. 4, 2006, pp. 663–676.

Ocampo, A. et al. 'In Vivo Amelioration of Age-Associated Hallmarks by Partial Reprogramming', *Cell*, vol. 167, no. 7, 2016, pp. 1719–1733.

Shen, J., Tsai, Y., Dimarco, N., Long, M., Sun, X., Tang, L. 'Transplantation of mesenchymal stem cells from young donors delays aging in mice', *Scientific Reports* vol. 1, no. 67, 2011.

Charles-de-Sá, L. et al. 'Photoaged Skin Therapy with Adipose-Derived Stem Cells', Plastic & Reconstructive Surgery, vol. 145, no. 6, 2020, pp. 1037e–1049e.

Xu, M. et al. 'Transplanted Senescent Cells Induce an Osteoarthritis-Like Condition in Mice', *The Journals of Gerontology, Series A: Biological Sciences and Medical Sciences*, vol. 72, no. 6, 2017, pp. 780–785.

Baker, D. et al. 'Naturally occurring p16 Ink4a-positive cells shorten healthy lifespan', *Nature*, vol. 530, no. 7589, 2016, pp. 184–189.

Xu, M., Pirtskhalava, T., Farr, J.N. 'Senolytics improve physical function and increase lifespan in old age', *Nature Medicine*, vol. 24, 2018, pp. 1246–1256.

Coppé, J., Patil, C. et al. 'Senescence-associated secretory phenotypes reveal cell-nonautonomous functions of oncogenic RAS and the p53 tumor suppressor', *PLOS Biology*, vol. 6, no. 12, 2008.

Muñoz-Espín, D. et al. 'Programmed cell senescence during mammalian embryonic development', *Cell*, vol. 155, no. 5, 2013, p. 1104.

Demaria, M. et al. 'An essential role for senescent cells in optimal wound healing through secretion of PDGF-AA', *Developmental Cell*, vol. 31, no. 6, 2014, pp. 722–733.

Cole, L., Kramer, P. *Apoptosis, Growth, and Aging*, Elsevier, 2016, pp. 63–66.

Spindler, S., Mote, P., Flegal, J., Teter, B. 'Influence on Longevity of Blueberry, Cinnamon, Green and Black Tea, Pomegranate, Sesame, Curcumin, Morin, Pycnogenol, Quercetin, and Taxifolin Fed Iso-Calorically to Long-Lived, F1 Hybrid Mice', *Rejuvenation Research*, vol. 16, no. 2, 2013, pp. 143–151.

Yousefzadeh, M. et al. 'Fisetin is a senotherapeutic that extends health and lifespan', *eBio Medicine*, vol. 36, 2018, pp. 18–28.

Xu, Q. et al. 'The flavonoid procyanidin C1 has senotherapeutic activity and increases lifespan in mice', *Nature Metabolism*, vol. 3, 2021, pp. 1706–1726.

Latorre, E., Torregrossa, R., Wood, M., Whiteman, M., Harries, L. 'Mitochondria-targeted hydrogen sulfide attenuates endothelial senescence by selective induction of splicing factors HNRNPD and SRSF2', *Aging*, vol. 10, no. 7, 2018, pp. 1666–1681.

'Unity biotechnology announces positive data from phase 1 clinical trial of ubx1325 in patients with advanced vascular eye disease', Unity Biotechnology Inc., 2021.

Wu, W., Li, R., Li, X., He, J., Jiang, S., Liu, S., Yang, J. 'Quercetin as an antiviral agent inhibits influenza a virus (IAV) Entry', *Viruses*, vol. 8, no. 1, 2015.

Chapter 12: Winding the Biological Clock

Horvath, S. 'DNA methylation age of human tissues and cell types', *Genome Biology*, vol. 14, no. 10, 2013, pp. 1–20.

Christiansen, L., Lenart, A., Tan, Q., Vaupel, J., Aviv, A., McGue, M., Christensen, K. 'DNA methylation age is associated with mortality in a longitudinal Danish twin study', *Aging Cell*, vol. 15, no. 1, 2016, pp. 149–154.

Marioni, R. et al. 'The epigenetic clock is correlated with physical and cognitive fitness in the Lothian Birth Cohort 1936', *International Journal of Epidemiology*, vol. 44, no. 4, 2015, pp. 1388–1396.

Horvath, S. et al. 'Decreased epigenetic age of PBMCs from Italian semi-supercentenarians and their offspring', *Aging*, vol. 7, no. 12, 2015, pp. 1159–1170.

Lu, A.T. et al. 'Universal DNA methylation age across mammalian tissues', bioRxiv, 2021. doi: https://doi. org/10.1101/2021.01.18. 426733

Horvath, S. et al. 'An epigenetic clock analysis of race/ethnicity, sex, and coronary heart disease', *Genome Biology*, vol. 17, no. 1, 2016, p. 171310.

Sehl, M., Henry, J., Storniolo, A., Ganz, P., Horvath, S. 'DNA methylation age is elevated in breast tissue of healthy women', *Breast Cancer Research and Treatment*, vol. 164, no. 1, pp. 209–219.

Kresovich, J., Xu, Z., O'Brien, K., Weinberg, C., Sandler, D., Taylor, J. 'Methylation-Based Biological Age and Breast Cancer Risk', *JNCI: Journal of the National Cancer Institute,* vol. 111, no. 10, 2019, pp. 1051–1058.

Horvath, S. et al. 'The cerebellum ages slowly according to the epigenetic clock', *Aging*, vol. 7, no. 5, 2017, pp. 294–306.

Dosi, R., Bhatt, N., Shah, P., Patell, R. 'Cardiovascular disease and menopause', *Journal of Clinical and Diagnostic Research*, vol. 8, no. 2, 2014, pp. 62–64.

Ossewaarde, M. et al. 'Age at menopause, cause-specific mortality and total life expectancy', *Epidemiology*, vol. 16, no. 4, 2005, pp. 556–562.

'The Nobel Prize in Physiology or Medicine 2016', NobelPrize.org, 2020.

Takahashi, K., Yamanaka, S. 'Induction of Pluripotent Stem Cells from Mouse Embryonic and Adult Fibroblast Cultures by Defined Factors', *Cell*, vol. 126, no. 4, 2006, pp. 663–676.

Ocampo, A. et al. 'In Vivo Amelioration of Age-Associated Hallmarks by Partial Reprogramming', *Cell*, vol. 167, no. 7, 2016, pp. 1719–1733.

Lu, Y., Brommer, B., Tian, X. et al. Reprogramming to recover youthful epigenetic information and restore vision. *Nature*, vol. 588, 2020, pp.124–129. https://doi.org/10.1038/s41586-020-2975-4

Shen, J., Tsai, Y., Dimarco, N., Long, M., Sun, X., Tang, L. 'Transplantation of mesenchymal stem cells from young donors delays aging in mice', *Scientific Reports*, vol. 1, no. 67, 2011.

Charles-de-Sá, L. et al. 'Photoaged Skin Therapy with Adipose-Derived Stem Cells', *Plastic & Reconstructive Surgery*, vol, 145, no. 6, pp. 1037e–1049e.

Kolata, G. 'A Cure for Type 1 Diabetes? For One Man, It Seems to Have Worked', *New York Times*, 2021.

Chapter 13: Bloody Marvellous

Huestis, D. 'Alexander Bogdanov: The Forgotten Pioneer of Blood Transfusion', *Transfusion Medicine Reviews*, vol. 21, no. 4, 2007, pp. 337–340.

Conboy, M., Conboy, I., Rando, T. 'Heterochronic parabiosis: Historical perspective and methodological considerations for studies of aging and longevity', *Aging Cell*, vol. 12, no. 3, 2013, pp. 525–530.

McCay, C., Pope, F., Lunsford, W., Sperling, G., Sambhavaphol, P. 'Parabiosis between Old and Young Rats', *Gerontology*, vol. 1, no. 1, 1957, pp. 7–17.

Conboy, I., Conboy, M., Wagers, A., Girma, E., Weismann, I., Rando, T. 'Rejuvenation of aged progenitor cells by exposure to a young systemic environment', *Nature*, vol. 433, no. 7027, 2005, pp. 760–764.

Villeda, S. et al. 'The ageing systemic milieu negatively regulates neurogenesis and cognitive function', *Nature*, vol. 477, no. 7362, 2011, pp. 90–96.

Mehdipour, M. et al. 'Rejuvenation of three germ layers tissues by exchanging old blood plasma with saline-albumin', *Aging*, vol. 12, no. 10, 2020, pp. 8790–8819.

Ullum, H. et al. 'Blood donation and blood donor mortality after adjustment for a healthy donor effect', *Transfusion*, vol. 55, no. 10, 2015, pp. 2479–2485.

Timmers, P. et al. 'Multivariate genomic scan implicates novel loci and haem metabolism in human ageing', *Nature Communications*, vol. 11, no. 3570, 2020.

Daghlas, I., Gill, D. 'Genetically predicted iron status and life expectancy', *Clinical Nutrition*, vol. 40, no. 4, 2020, pp. 2456–2459.

Kadoglou, N., Biddulph, J., Rafnsson, S., Trivella, M., Nihoyannopoulos, P., Demakakos, P. 'The association of ferritin with cardiovascular and all-cause mortality in community-dwellers: The English longitudinal study of ageing', *PLOS ONE*, vol. 12, no. 6, 2017.

Forte, G. et al. 'Metals in plasma of nonagenarians and centenarians living in a key area of longevity', *Experimental Gerontology*, vol. 60, 2014, pp. 197–206.

Ford, E., Cogswell, M. 'Diabetes and serum ferritin concentration among U.S. adults', *Diabetes Care*, vol. 22, no. 12, 1999, pp. 1978–1983.

Tuomainen, T. et al. 'Body iron stores are associated with serum insulin and blood glucose concentrations: Population study in 1,013 eastern Finnish men', *Diabetes Care*, vol. 20, no. 3, 1997, pp. 426–428.

Bonfils, L. et al. 'Fasting serum levels of ferritin are associated with impaired pancreatic beta cell function and decreased insulin sensitivity: a population-based study', *Diabetologia*, vol. 58, no. 3, 2015, pp. 523–533.

Zacharski, L. et al. 'Decreased cancer risk after iron reduction in patients with peripheral arterial disease: Results from a randomized trial', *Journal of the National Cancer Institute*, vol. 100, no. 14, 2008, pp. 996–1002.

Mursu, J., Robien, K., Harnack, L., Park, K., Jacobs, D. 'Dietary supplements and mortality rate in older women: The Iowa Women's Health Study', *Archives of Internal Medicine*, vol. 171, no. 18, 2011, pp. 1625–1633.

Kell, D., Pretorius, E. 'No effects without causes: the Iron Dysregulation and Dormant Microbes hypothesis for chronic, inflammatory diseases' *Biological Reviews*, vol. 93, no. 3, 2018, pp. 1518–1557.

Parmanand, B., Kellingray, L. et al. 'A decrease in iron availability to human gut microbiome reduces the growth of potentially pathogenic gut bacteria; an in vitro colonic fermentation study', *Journal of Nutritional Biochemistry*, vol. 67, 2019, pp. 20–22.

Ayton, S. et al. 'Brain iron is associated with accelerated cognitive decline in people with Alzheimer pathology', *Molecular Psychiatry*, vol. 25, 2020, pp. 2932–2941.

Cross, J. et al. 'Oral iron acutely elevates bacterial growth in human serum', *Scientific Reports*, vol. 5, no. 16670, 2015.

Semenova, E.A. et al. 'The association of HFE gene H63D polymorphism with endurance athlete status and aerobic capacity: novel findings and a meta-analysis', *Eur J Appl Physiol.*, vol. 120, no. 3, 2020, pp. 665–673. doi: 10.1007/s00421-020-04306-8.

Thakkar, D., Sicova, M., Guest, N.S., Garcia-Bailo, B., El-Sohemy, A. 'HFE Genotype and Endurance Performance in Competitive Male Athletes', *Med Sci Sports Exerc.*, vol. 53, no. 7, 2021, pp. 1385–1390. doi: 10.1249/MSS.0000000000002595.

Chapter 14: Microbe Struggles

Zoltán, I. 'Ignaz Semmelweis', *Encyclopaedia Britannica*, 2020, www.britannica.com/biography/Ignaz-Semmelweis.

Levy, C. 'De nyeste Forsög i Födselsstiftelsen i Wien til Oplysning om Barselsfeberens Ætiologie', Hospitals-Meddelelser, *Tidskrift for praktisk Lægevidenskab*, vol. 1, 1848.

Kidd, M., Modlin, I. 'A Century of *Helicobacter pylori*', *Digestion*, vol. 59, 1998, pp. 1–15.

Phillips, M. 'John Lykoudis and peptic ulcer disease', *Lancet*, vol. 255, no. 9198, 2000.

'The Nobel Prize in Physiology or Medicine 2005', NobelPrize.org, 2020.

Sender, R., Fuchs, S., Milo, R. 'Are we really outnumbered? Revisiting the ratio of bacterial to host cells in humans', *Cell*, vol. 164, no. 3, 2016, pp. 337–340.

Scheiman, J. et al. 'Meta-omics analysis of elite athletes identifies a performance-enhancing microbe that functions via lactate metabolism', *Nature Medicine*, vol. 25, 2019, pp. 1104–1109.

Damgaard, C. et al. 'Viable bacteria associated with red blood cells and plasma in freshly drawn blood donations', *PLOS ONE*, vol. 10, no. 3, 2015.

Servick, K. 'Do gut bacteria make a second home in our brains?', www.science.org, 9 November 2018.

Beros, S., Lenhart, A., Scharf, I., Negroni, M.A., Menzel, F., Foitzik, S. 'Extreme lifespan extension in tapeworm-infected ant workers', *Royal Society Open Science*, vol. 8, no. 5, 2021. https://doi.org/10.1098/rsos.202118.

Chapter 15: Hiding in Plain Sight

Mina, M., Metcalf, C., De Swart, R., Osterhaus, A., Grenfell, B. 'Infectious Disease Mortality', *Science*, vol. 348, no. 6235, 2015, pp 694–699.

Powell, M. et al. 'Opportunistic infections in HIV-infected patients differ strongly in frequencies and spectra between patients with low CD4+ cell counts examined postmortem and compensated patients examined antemortem irrespective of the HAART Era', *PLOS ONE*, vol. 11, no. 9, 2016.

Horvath, S., Levine, A. 'HIV-1 Infection Accelerates Age According to the Epigenetic Clock', *Journal of Infectious Diseases*, vol. 212, no. 10, 2015, pp. 1563–1571.

Fülöp, T., Larbi, A., Pawelec, G. 'Human T-cell aging and the impact of persistent viral infections', *Frontiers in Immunology*, vol. 4, 2013, p. 271.

Sylwester, A. et al. 'Broadly targeted human cytomegalovirus-specific CD4+ and CD8+ T-cells dominate the memory compartments of exposed subjects', *Journal of Experimental Medicine*, vol. 202, no. 5, 2005, pp. 673–685.

Cheng, J., Ke, Q. et al. 'Cytomegalovirus infection causes an increase of arterial blood pressure', *PLOS Pathogens*, vol. 5, no. 5, 2009, p. 1000427.

Goldmacher, V. 'Cell death suppression by cytomegaloviruses', *Apoptosis*, vol. 10, no. 2, March 2005, pp. 251–265.

Aguilera, M., Delgui, L., Romano, P., Colombo, M. 'Chronic Infections: A Possible Scenario for Autophagy and Senescence Cross-Talk', *Cells*, vol. 7, no. 10, 2018, p. 162.

Revello, M., Gerna, G. 'Diagnosis and management of human cytomegalovirus infection in the mother, fetus, and newborn infant', *Clinical Microbiology Reviews*, vol. 15, no. 4, 2002, pp. 680–715.

Bjornevik, K., Cortese, M. et al. 'Longitudinal analysis reveals high prevalence of Epstein-Barr virus associated with multiple sclerosis', *Science*, vol. 375, no. 6578, 2022, pp. 296–301.

Harvey, E.M., McNeer, E., McDonald, M.F. et al. 'Association of Preterm Birth Rate With COVID-19 Statewide Stay-at-Home Orders in Tennessee', *JAMA Pediatr.*, vol. 175, no. 6, 2021, pp. 635–637. doi:10.1001/jamapediatrics.2020.6512.

Crist, C. 'COVID-19 May Raise Risk of Diabetes in Children', *WebMD*, 2022.

Chapter 16: Flossing for Longevity

Soscia, S. et al. 'The Alzheimer's Disease-Associated Amyloid β-Protein Is an Antimicrobial Peptide', *PLOS ONE*, vol. 5, no. 3, 2010, e9505.

Kumar, D. et al. 'Amyloid-β peptide protects against microbial infection in mouse and worm models of Alzheimer's disease', *Science Translational Medicine*, vol. 8, no. 340, 2016.

Lambert, J. et al. 'Meta-analysis of 74,046 individuals identifies 11 new susceptibility loci for Alzheimer's disease', *Nature Genetics*, vol. 45, no. 12, 2013, pp. 1452–1458.

Itzhaki, R. 'Corroboration of a Major Role for Herpes Simplex Virus Type 1 in Alzheimer's Disease', *Frontiers in Aging Neuroscience*, vol. 10, no. 324, 2018.

Tzeng, N. et al. 'Anti-herpetic Medications and Reduced Risk of Dementia in Patients with Herpes Simplex Virus Infections—a Nationwide, Population-Based Cohort Study in Taiwan', *Neurotherapeutics*, vol. 15, no. 2, 2018, pp. 417–429.

Wozniak, M., Itzhaki, R., Shipley, S., Dobson, C. 'Herpes simplex virus infection causes cellular β-amyloid accumulation and secretase up-regulation', *Neuroscience Letters*, vol. 429, no. 2–3, 2007, pp. 95–100.

Wozniak, M., Frost, A., Preston, C., Itzhaki, R. 'Antivirals reduce the formation of key Alzheimer's disease molecules in cell cultures acutely infected with herpes simplex virus type 1', *PLOS ONE*, vol. 6, no. 10, 2011.

Wozniak, M., Mee, A., Itzhaki, R. 'Herpes simplex virus type 1 DNA is located within Alzheimer's disease amyloid plaques', *Journal of Pathology*, vol. 217, no. 1, 2009, pp. 131–138.

Dominy, S. et al. 'Porphyromonas gingivalis in Alzheimer's disease brains: Evidence for disease causation and treatment with small-molecule inhibitors', *Science Advances*, vol. 5, no. 1, 2019.

Demmer, R. et al. 'Periodontal disease and incident dementia: The Atherosclerosis Risk in Communities Study (ARIC)', *Neurology*, vol. 95, no. 12, 2020, pp. e1660– e1671.

Bui, F. et al. 'Association between periodontal pathogens and systemic disease', *Biomedical Journal,* vol. 42, no. 1, 2019, pp. 27–35.

Balin, B. et al. 'Chlamydophila pneumoniae and the etiology of late-onset Alzheimer's disease', *Journal of Alzheimer's Disease*, vol. 13, no. 4, 2008, pp. 371–380.

Balin, B. et al. 'Identification and localization of Chlamydia pneumoniae in the Alzheimer's brain', *Medical Microbiology and Immunology*, vol. 187, no. 1, 1998, pp. 23–42.

Pisa, D., Alonso, R., Rábano, A., Rodal, I., Carrasco, L. 'Different Brain Regions are Infected with Fungi in Alzheimer's Disease', *Scientific Reports*, vol. 5, no. 1, 2015, pp. 1–13.

Wu, Y. 'Microglia and amyloid precursor protein coordinate control of transient *Candida cerebritis* with memory deficits', *Nature Communications*, vol. 10, no. 58, 2019.

Edrey, Y., Medina, D. et al. 'Amyloid beta and the longest-lived rodent: The naked mole-rat as a model for natural protection from Alzheimer's disease', *Neurobiology of Aging*, vol. 34, no. 10, 2013, pp. 2352–2360.

Steinmann, G., Klaus, B., Müller-Hermelink, H. 'The Involution of the Ageing Human Thymic Epithelium is Independent of Puberty: A Morphometric Study', *Scandinavian Journal of Immunology*, vol. 22, no. 5, 1985, pp. 563–575.

Kulikov, A., Arkhipova, L., Kulikov, D., Smirnova, G., Kulikova, P. 'The increase of the average and maximum span of life by the allogenic thymic cells transplantation in the animals' anterior chamber of eye', *Advances in Gerontology*, vol. 4, no. 3, 2014, pp. 197–200.

Oh, J., Wang, W., Thomas, R., Su, D. 'Thymic rejuvenation via induced thymic epithelial cells (iTECs) from FOXN1 -overexpressing fibroblasts to counteract inflammaging', *BioRxiv*, 2020.

Weiss, R., Vogt, P. '100 years of Rous sarcoma virus', *Journal of Experimental Medicine*, vol. 208, no. 12, 2011, pp. 2351–2355.

'The Nobel Prize in Physiology or Medicine 1966', NobelPrize.org, 2020.

White, M., Pagano, J., Khalili, K. 'Viruses and human cancers: A long road of discovery of molecular paradigms', *Clinical Microbiology Reviews*, vol. 27, no. 3, 2014, pp. 463–471.

Gillison, M. 'Human Papillomavirus-Related Diseases: Oropharynx Cancers and Potential Implications for Adolescent HPV Vaccination', *Journal of Adolescent Health*, vol. 43, no. 4 , 2008, pp. S52–S60.

Bzhalava, D., Guan, P., Franceschi, S., Dillner, J., Clifford, G. 'A systematic review of the prevalence of mucosal and cutaneous Human Papillomavirus types', *Virology*, vol. 445, no. 1–2, 2013, pp. 224–231.

Nejman, D. et al. 'The human tumor microbiome is composed of tumor type-specific intracellular bacteria', *Science*, vol. 368, no. 6494, 2020, pp. 973–980.

Bullman, S. et al. 'Analysis of Fusobacterium persistence and antibiotic response in colorectal cancer', *Science*, vol. 358, no. 6369, 2017, pp. 1443–1448.

Aykut, B. 'The fungal mycobiome promotes pancreatic oncogenesis via activation of MBL', *Nature*, vol. 574, no. 7777, 2019, pp. 264–267.

Michalek, A., Mettlin, C., Priore, R. 'Prostate cancer mortality among Catholic priests', *Journal of Surgical Oncology*, vol. 17, no. 2, 1981, pp. 129–133.

Shah, P. 'Link between infection and atherosclerosis: Who are the culprits: Viruses, bacteria, both, or neither?', *Circulation*, vol. 103, 2001, pp. 5–6.

Haraszthy, V., Zambon, J., Trevisan, M., Zeid, M., Genco, R. 'Identification of Periodontal Pathogens in Atheromatous Plaques', *Journal of Periodontology*, vol. 71, no. 10, 2000, pp. 1554–1560.

Warren-Gash, C., Blackburn, R., Whitaker, H., McMenamin, J., Hayward, A. 'Laboratory-confirmed respiratory infections as triggers for acute myocardial infarction and stroke: A self-controlled case series analysis of national linked datasets from Scotland', *European Respiratory Journal*, vol. 51, no. 3, 2018.

Anand, S., Tikoo, S. 'Viruses as modulators of mitochondrial functions', *Advances in Virology*, vol. 2013, 2013, 738794.

Wang, C., Youle, R. 'The role of mitochondria in apoptosis', *Annual Review of Genetics*, vol. 43, 2009, pp. 95–118.

Choi, Y., Bowman, J., Jung, J. 'Autophagy during viral infection – A double-edged sword', *Nature Reviews Microbiology*, vol. 16, 2018, pp. 341–354.

Sudhakar, P. et al. 'Targeted interplay between bacterial pathogens and host autophagy', *Autophagy*, vol. 15, no. 9, 2019, pp. 1620–1633.

Li, M., MacDonald, M. 'Polyamines: Small Molecules with a Big Role in Promoting Virus Infection', *Cell Host & Microbe*, vol. 20, no. 2, 2016, pp. 123–124.

Altindis, E. et al. 'Viral insulin-like peptides activate human insulin and IGF-1 receptor signaling: A paradigm shift for host–microbe interactions', *Proceedings of the National Academy of Sciences of the United States of America*, vol. 115, no. 10, 2018, pp. 2461–2466.

Liu, Y. et al. 'The extracellular domain of Staphylococcus aureus LtaS binds insulin and induces insulin resistance during infection', *Nature Microbiology*, vol. 3, 2018, pp. 622–31.

Chang, F.Y., Siuti, P., Laurent, S. et al. 'Gut-inhabiting Clostridia build human GPCR ligands by conjugating neurotransmitters with diet- and human-derived fatty acids', *Nat Microbiol.*, 2021, vol. 6, pp. 792–805. https://doi.org/10.1038/s41564-021-00887-y.

Chapter 17: Immune Rejuvenation

Smith, P., Willemsen, D. et al. 'Regulation of life span by the gut microbiota in the short-lived African turquoise killifish,' *eLife* vol. 6, 2017.

Kundu, P. et al. 'Neurogenesis and prolongevity signaling in young germ-free mice transplanted with the gut microbiota of old mice', *Science Translational Medicine*, vol. 11, no. 518, 2019, p. 4760.

Aleman, F., Valenzano, D. 'Microbiome evolution during host aging', *PLOS Pathogens*, vol. 15, no. 7, 2019.

Yousefzadeh, M.J., Flores, R.R., Zhu, Y. et al. 'An aged immune system drives senescence and ageing of solid organs', *Nature*, vol. 594, 2021, pp. 100–105. https://doi.org/10.1038/s41586-021-03547-7.

Campinoti, S., Gjinovci, A., Ragazzini, R. et al. 'Reconstitution of a functional human thymus by postnatal stromal progenitor cells and natural whole-organ scaffolds', *Nat Commun.*, vol. 11: 6372, 2020. https://doi.org/10.1038/s41467-020-20082-7.

Franceschi, C. et al. 'Inflammaging and anti-inflammaging: A systemic perspective on aging and longevity emerged from studies in humans,' *Mechanisms of Ageing and Development*, vol. 128, no. 1, 2007, pp. 92–105.

Chapter 18: Starving for Fun

McCay, C., Crowell, M., Maynard, L. 'The effect of retarded growth upon the length of life span and upon the ultimate body size', *The Journal of Nutrition,* vol. 10, no. 1, July 1935, pp. 63–79.

Schäfer, D. 'Aging, Longevity, and Diet: Historical Remarks on Calorie Intake Reduction', *Gerontology*, vol. 51, no. 2, 2005, pp. 126–130.

McDonald, R. Ramsey, J. 'Honoring Clive McCay and 75 years of calorie restriction research', *Journal of Nutrition*, vol. 140, no. 7, 2010, pp. 1205–1210.

Weindruch, R., Walford, R. 'Dietary restriction in mice beginning at 1 year of age: Effect on life span and spontaneous cancer incidence', *Science*, vol. 215, no. 4538, 1982, pp. 1415–1418.

Weindruch, R., Walford, R., Fligiel, S., Guthrie, D. 'The retardation of aging in mice by dietary restriction: Longevity, cancer, immunity and lifetime energy intake', *Journal of Nutrition*, vol. 116, no. 4, 1986, pp. 641–654.

Walford, R., Mock, D., Verdery, R., MacCallum, T.J. 'Calorie restriction in Biosphere 2: Alterations in physiologic, hematologic, hormonal, and biochemical parameters in humans restricted for a 2-year period', *The Journals of Gerontology, Series A: Biological Sciences and Medical Sciences*, vol. 57, no. 6, 2002, pp. B211–B224.

Mattison, J. et al. 'Caloric restriction improves health and survival of rhesus monkeys', *Nature Communications*, vol. 8, no. 14063, 2017.

Colman, R., Anderson, R. et al. 'Caloric restriction delays disease onset and mortality in rhesus monkeys', *Science*, vol. 325, no. 5937, 2009, pp. 201–204.

Mattison, J. et al. 'Impact of caloric restriction on health and survival in rhesus monkeys from the NIA study', *Nature*, vol. 489, no. 7415, 2012, pp. 318–321.

Kraus, W. et al. '2 years of calorie restriction and cardiometabolic risk (CALERIE): exploratory outcomes of a multicentre, phase 2, randomised controlled trial', *The Lancet Diabetes and Endocrinology*, vol. 7, no. 9, 2019, pp. 673–683.

Jia, K., Levine, B. 'Autophagy is required for dietary restriction-mediated life span extension in *C. elegans*', *Autophagy*, vol. 3, no.6, 2007, pp. 597–599.

Saxton, R., Sabatini, D. 'mTOR Signaling in Growth, Metabolism, and Disease', *Cell*, vol. 168, no. 6, 2017, pp. 960–976.

Chapter 19: An Old Custom in New Clothes

Di Francesco, A., Di Germanio, C., Bernier, M., De Cabo, R. 'A time to fast', *Science*, vol. 362, no. 6416, 2018, pp. 770–775.

Michael Anson, R. et al. 'Intermittent fasting dissociates beneficial effects of dietary restriction on glucose metabolism and neuronal resistance to injury from calorie intake', *Proceedings of the National Academy of Sciences of the United States of America*, vol. 100, no. 10, 2003, pp. 6216–6220.

Mitchell, S. et al. 'Daily Fasting Improves Health and Survival in Male Mice Independent of Diet Composition and Calories', *Cell Metabolism*, vol. 29, no. 1, 2019, pp. 221–228.

Woodie, L., Luo, Y., et al. 'Restricted feeding for 9 h in the active period partially abrogates the detrimental metabolic effects of a Western diet with liquid sugar consumption in mice', *Metabolism: Clinical and Experimental*, vol. 82, 2018, pp. 1–13.

Carlson, A., Hoelzel, F. 'Apparent prolongation of the life span of rats by intermittent fasting', *The Journal of Nutrition*, vol. 31, no. 3, 1946, pp. 363–375.

Wei, M. et al. 'Fasting-mimicking diet and markers/risk factors for aging, diabetes, cancer, and cardiovascular disease', *Science Translational Medicine*, vol. 9, no. 377, 2017.

Stewart, W., Fleming, L. 'Features of a successful therapeutic fast of 382 days' duration', *Postgraduate Medical Journal*, vol. 49, no. 569, 1973, pp. 203–209.

Heilbronn, L., Smith, S., Martin, C., Anton, S., Ravussin, E. 'Alternate-day fasting in non-obese subjects: effects on body weight, body composition, and energy metabolism', *The American Journal of Clinical Nutrition*, vol. 81, no. 1, 2005, pp. 69–73.

Tinsley, G., Forsse, J. et al. 'Time-restricted feeding in young men performing resistance training: A randomized controlled trial', *European Journal of Sport Science*, vol. 17, no. 2, 2017, pp. 200–207.

Fillmore, K., Stockwell, T., Chikritzhs, T., Bostrom, A., Kerr, W. 'Moderate Alcohol Use and Reduced Mortality Risk: Systematic Error in Prospective Studies and New Hypotheses', *Annals of Epidemiology*, vol. 17, no. 5, 2007, pp. S16–S23.

Burton, R., Sheron, N. 'No level of alcohol consumption improves health', *Lancet*, vol. 392, no. 10152, 2018, pp. 987–988.

Kim, Y., Je, Y., Giovannucci, E. 'Coffee consumption and all-cause and cause-specific mortality: a meta-analysis by potential modifiers', *European Journal of Epidemiology*, vol. 34, 2019, pp. 731–752.

Freedman, N., Park, Y., Abnet, C., Hollenbeck, A., Sinha, R. 'Association of Coffee Drinking with Total and Cause-Specific Mortality', *New England Journal of Medicine*, vol. 366, 2012, pp. 1891–1904.

Chapter 20: Cargo Cult Nutrition

Bianconi, E. et al. 'An estimation of the number of cells in the human body', *Annals of Human Biology*, vol. 40, no. 6, 2013, pp. 463–471.

OECD. 'Life expectancy by sex and education level', *Health at a Glance 2017: OECD Indicators*, OECD Publishing, 2017. https://doi.org/10.1787/health_glance-2017-7-en.

Brønnum-Hansen, H., Baadsgaard, M. 'Widening social inequality in life expectancy in Denmark. A register-based study on social composition and mortality trends for the Danish population', *BMC Public Health*, vol. 12, no. 994, 2012.

Hummer, R.A., Hernandez, E.M. 'The Effect of Educational Attainment on Adult Mortality in the United States', *Popul Bull*, vol. 68, no. 1, 2013, pp. 1–16.

Fraser, G. 'Vegetarian diets: What do we know of their effects on common chronic diseases?' *American Journal of Clinical Nutrition*, vol. 89, no. 5, 2009, pp. 1607S–1612S.

Mihrshahi, S., Ding, D. et al. 'Vegetarian diet and all-cause mortality: Evidence from a large population-based Australian cohort – the 45 and Up Study', *Preventive Medicine*, vol. 97, 2017, pp. 1–7.

Zhao, L.G., Sun, J.W., Yang, Y. et al. 'Fish consumption and all-cause mortality: a meta-analysis of cohort studies', *Eur J Clin Nutr.*, vol. 70, 2016, pp. 155–161.

Zhang, Y., Zhuang, P, He, W. et al. 'Association of fish and long-chain omega-3 fatty acids intakes with total and cause-specific mortality: prospective analysis of 421 309 individuals', *JIM*, vol. 284, no. 4, 2018, pp. 399–417.

McBurney, M.I., Tintle, N., Ramachandran, S.V., Sala-Vila, A., Harris, W.S. 'Using an erythrocyte fatty acid fingerprint to predict risk of all-cause mortality: the Framingham Offspring Cohort', *The American Journal of Clinical Nutrition*, vol. 114, no. 4, 2021, pp.1447–1454.

Harris, W.S., Tintle, N.L. et al. 'Blood n-3 fatty acid levels and total and cause-specific mortality from 17 prospective studies', *Nature Communications*, vol. 12: 2329, 2021.

Bernasconi, A.A., Wiest, M.M., Lavie, C.J., Milani, R.V., Laukkanen, J.A. 'Effect of Omega-3 Dosage on Cardiovascular Outcomes: An Updated meta-Analysis and Meta-Regression of Interventional Trials', *Mayo Clinic Proceedings*, vol. 96, no. 2, 2021, pp. 304–313.

Cawthorn, D-M., Baillie, C., Mariani, S. 'Generic names and mislabelling conceal high species diversity in global fisheries markets', *Conservation Letters*, vol. 11, no. 5, 2018, p. e12573.

Willette, D.A., Simmonds, S.E., Cheng, S.H. et al. 'Using DNA barcoding to track seafood mislabelling in Los Angeles restaurants', *Conservation Biology*, vol. 31, no. 5, 2017, pp. 1076–1085.

Ho, J.K.I., Puniamoorthy, J., Srivathsan, A., Meier, R. 'MinION sequencing of seafood in Singapore reveals creatively labelled flatfishes, confused roe, pig DNA in squid balls, and phantom crustaceans', *Food Control*, vol. 112, 2020, p. 107144.

Autier, P., Boniol, M., Pizot, C., Mullie, P. 'Vitamin D status and ill health: a systematic review', *The Lancet: Diabetes & Endocrinology*, vol. 2, no. 1, 2014, pp. 76–90.

Lin, S., Jiang, L., Zhang, Y., Chai, J., Li, J., Song, X., Pei, L. 'Soci-oeconomic status and vitamin D deficiency among women of childbearing age: a population-based, case-control study in rural northern China', *BMJ Open*, vol. 11, 2021, p. e042227.

Zhang, Y., Fang, F., Tang, J., Jia, L., Feng, Y., Xu, P. et al. 'Association between vitamin D supplementation and mortality: systematic review and meta-analysis', *BMJ*, vol. 366, 2019, p. 14673. doi:10.1136/bmj.l4673.

Chapter 21: Food for Thought

Perry, G. et al. 'Diet and the evolution of human amylase gene copy number variation', *Nature Genetics*, vol. 39, no. 10, 2007, pp. 1256–1260.

Arendt, M., Cairns, K., Ballard, J., Savolainen, P., Axelsson, E. 'Diet adaptation in dog reflects spread of prehistoric agriculture', *Heredity*, vol. 117, no. 5, 2016, pp. 301–306

Ségurel, L., Bon, C. 'On the Evolution of Lactase Persistence in Humans', *Annual Review of Genomics and Human Genetics*, vol. 18, 2017, pp. 297–319.

Gross, M. 'How our diet changed our evolution', *Current Biology*, vol. 27, no. 15, 2017, pp. 731–733.

Chapter 22: Medieval Monks to Modern Science

Kenyon, C., Chang, J., Gensch, E., Rudner, A., Tabtiang, R. 'A C. elegans mutant that lives twice as long as wild type', *Nature*, vol. 366, no. 6454, 1993, pp. 461–464.

Wijsman, C. et al. 'Familial longevity is marked by enhanced insulin sensitivity', *Aging Cell*, vol. 10, no. 1, 2011, pp. 114–121.

Yashin, A., Arbeev, K. et al. 'Exceptional survivors have lower age trajectories of blood glucose: Lessons from longitudinal data', *Biogerontology*, vol. 11, no. 3, 2010, pp. 257–265.

Kurosu, H. et al. 'Physiology: Suppression of aging in mice by the hormone Klotho', *Science*, vol. 309, no. 5742, 2005, pp. 1829–1833.

Lindeberg, S., Eliasson, M., Lindahl, B., Ahrén, B. 'Low serum insulin in traditional Pacific islanders – The Kitava study', *Metabolism: Clinical and Experimental*, vol. 48, no. 10, 1999, pp. 1216–1219.

Li, H., Gao, Z. et al. 'Sodium butyrate stimulates expression of fibroblast growth factor 21 in liver by inhibition of histone deacetylase 3', *Diabetes*, vol. 61, no. 4, 2012, pp. 797–806.

Zhang, Y. et al. 'The starvation hormone, fibroblast growth factor-21, extends lifespan in mice', *eLife,* vol. 2012, no. 1, 2012.

Reynolds, A., Mann, J., Cummings, J., Winter, N., Mete, E., Te Morenga, L. 'Carbohydrate quality and human health: a series of systematic reviews and meta-analyses' *The Lancet*, vol. 393, no. 10170, 2019, pp. 434–445.

Buffenstein, R., Yahav, S. 'The effect of diet on microfaunal population and function in the caecum of a subterranean naked mole-rat, *Heterocephalus glaber*', *British Journal of Nutrition*, vol. 65, no. 2, 1991, pp. 249–258.

Al-Regaiey, K., Masternak, M., Bonkowski, M., Sun, L., Bartke, A. 'Long-Lived Growth Hormone Receptor Knockout Mice: Interaction of Reduced Insulin-Like Growth Factor I/Insulin Signaling and Caloric Restriction', *Endocrinology*, vol. 146, no. 2, 2005, pp. 851–860.

Zeevi, D., Korem, T., Zmora, N. et al. 'Personalized Nutrition by Prediction of Glycemic Responses', *Cell*, vol. 163, no. 5, 2015, pp. 2069–1094.

Frampton, J., Cobbold, B., Nozdrin, M. et al. 'The Effect of a Single Bout of Continuous Aerobic Exercise on Glucose, Insulin and Glucagon Concentrations Compared to resting Conditions in Healthy Adults: A Systematic Review, Meta-Analysis and Meta-Regression', *Sports Medicine*, vol. 51, 2021, pp. 1949–1966.

Solomon, T.P.J., Tarry, E., Hudson, C.O., Fitt, A.I., Laye, M.J. 'Immediate post-breakfast physical activity improves interstitial postprandial glycemia: a comparison of different activity-meal timings', *Pflugers Archiv – European Journal of Physiology*, vol. 572, 2020, pp. 271–280.

Bannister, C. et al. 'Can people with type 2 diabetes live longer than those without? A comparison of mortality in people initiated with metformin or sulphonylurea monotherapy and matched, non-diabetic controls', *Diabetes, Obesity and Metabolism*, vol. 16, no. 11, 2014, pp. 1165–1173.

Konopka, A. et al. 'Metformin inhibits mitochondrial adaptations to aerobic exercise training in older adults', *Aging Cell*, vol. 18, no. 1, 2019, p. 12880.

Walton, R. et al. 'Metformin blunts muscle hypertrophy in response to progressive resistance exercise training in older adults: A randomized, double-blind, placebo-controlled, multicenter trial: The MASTERS trial', *Aging Cell*, vol. 18, no. 6, 2019.

Chapter 23: What Gets Measured Gets Managed

Stary, H.C., Chandler, A.B., Glagov, S. et al. 'A definition of initial, fatty streak, and intermediate lesions of atherosclerosis. A report from the Committee on Vascular Lesions of the Council on Arteriosclerosis, American Heart Association', *Circulation*, vol. 89, no. 5, 1994, pp. 2462–2478.

Enos, W.F., Holmes, R.H., Beyer, J. 'Coronary disease among united states soldiers killed in action in korea', *JAMA*, vol. 152, no. 12, 1953, pp. 1090–1093. doi:10.1001/jama.1953.03690120006002.

Velican, D., Velican, C. 'Study of fibrous plaques occurring in the coronary arteries of children', *atherosclerosis*, vol. 33, no. 2, 1979, pp. 201–215.

Cohen, J., Pertsemlidis, A., Kotowski, I.K., Graham, R., Garcia, C.K., Hobbs, H.H. 'Low LDL cholesterol in individuals of African descent resulting from frequent nonsense mutations in PCSK9', *Nature Genetics*, vol. 37, 2005, pp. 161–165.

Kathiresan, S. 'A PCSK9 Missense Variant Associated with a Reduced Risk of Early-Onset Myocardial Infarction', *N Engl J Med.*, vol. 358, 2008, pp. 2299–2300. doi: 10.1056/NEJMc0707445.

Kent, S.T., Rosenson, R.S., Avery, C.L. et al. 'PCSK9 Loss-of-Function Variants, Low-Density Lipoprotein Cholesterol, and Risk of

Coronary Heart Disease and Stroke', *Circulation*, vol. 10, no. 4, 2017

Ference, B.A. et al. 'Low-density lipoproteins cause atherosclerotic cardiovascular disease. 1. Evidence from genetic, epidemiologic, and clinical studies. A consensus statement from the European Atherosclerosis Society Consensus Panel', *European Heart Journal*, vol. 38, no. 32, 2017, pp. 2459–2472.

Kern, F. Jr. 'Normal Plasma Cholesterol in an 88-Year-Old Man Who Eats 25 Eggs a Day – Mechanisms of Adaptation', *N Engl J Med.*, vol. 324, 1991, pp. 896–899. doi: 10.1056/ NEJM199103283241306.

Hirshowitz, B., Brook, J.G., Kaufman, T., Titelman, U., Mahler, D. '35 eggs per day in the treatment of severe burns,' *Br J Plast Surg.*, vol. 28, no. 3, 1975, pp. 185–188.

Kaufman, T., Hirshowitz, B., Moscona, R., Brook, G.J. 'Early enteral nutrition for mass burn injury: The revised egg-rich diet,' *Burns*, vol. 12, no. 4, 1986, pp. 260–263.

Drouin-Chartier, J., Chen, S., Li, Y., Schwab, A.L., Stamp-fer, M.J., Sacks, F.M. et al. 'Egg consumption and risk of cardio-vascular disease: three large prospective US cohort studies, sys-tematic review, and updated meta-nalysis', *BMJ*, 368:m513, 2020. doi:10.1136/bmj.m513.

Jones, P., Pappu, A., Hatcher, L., Li, Z., Illingworth, D., Connor, W. 'Dietary cholesterol feeding suppresses human cholesterol syn-thesis measured by deuterium incorporation and urinary meva-lonic acid levels', *Arteriosclerosis, Thrombosis, and Vascular Biology*, vol. 16, no. 10, 1996, pp. 1222–1228.

Steiner, M. Khan, A.H., Holbert, D., Lin, R.I. 'A double-blind crossover study in moderately hypercholesterolemic men that compared the effect of aged garlic extract and placebo admin-istration on blood lipids', *Am J Clin Nutr.*, vol. 64, no. 6, 1996, pp. 866–870. doi: 10.1093/ajcn/65.6.866.

Sobenin, I.A., Andrianova, I.V., Demidova, O.N., Gorchakova, T., Orekhov, A.N. 'Lipid-lowering effects of time-released garlic powder tablets in double-blinded placebo-controlled randomized study', *J Atheroscler Thromb.*, vol. 15, no. 6, 2008, pp. 334–338. doi: 10.5551/jat.e550.

McRae, M.P. 'Dietary Fiber is Beneficial for the Prevention of Cardiovascular Disease: An Umbrella Review of Meta-analyses', *Journal of Chiropractic Medicine*, vol. 16, no. 4, 2017, pp. 289–299.

Franco, O., Peeters, A., Bonneux, L., De Laet, C. 'Blood pressure in adulthood and life expectancy with cardiovascular disease in men and women: Life course analysis', *Hypertension*, vol. 46, no. 2, 2005, pp. 280–286.

Benigni, A. et al. 'Variations of the angiotensin II type 1 receptor gene are associated with extreme human longevity', *Age*, vol. 35, no. 3, 2013, pp. 993–1005.

Benigni, A. et al. 'Disruption of the Ang II type 1 receptor promotes longevity in mice', *Journal of Clinical Investigation*, vol. 119, no. 3, 2009, p. 52.

Basso, N., Cini, R., Pietrelli, A., Ferder, L., Terragno, N. Inserra, F. 'Protective effect of long-term angiotensin II inhibition', *American Journal of Physiology – Heart and Circulatory Physiology*, vol. 293, no. 3, 2007, pp. 1351–1358.

Kumar, S., Dietrich, N., Kornfeld, K. 'Angiotensin Converting Enzyme (ACE) Inhibitor Extends *Caenorhabditis elegans* Life Span', *PLOS Genetics*, vol. 12, no. 2, 2016.

Mueller, N., Noya-Alarcon, O., Contreras, M., Appel, L., Dominguez-Bello, M. 'Association of Age with Blood Pressure Across the Lifespan in Isolated Yanomami and Yekwana Villages', *JAMA Cardiology*, vol. 3, no. 12, 2018, pp. 1247–1249.

Lindeberg, S. *Food and Western Disease*, Wiley, 2009.

Gurven, M. et al. 'Does blood pressure inevitably rise with age? Longitudinal evidence among forager-horticulturalists', *Hypertension*, vol. 60, no. 1, 2012, pp. 25–33. doi: 10.1161/HYPERTENSIONAHA.111.189100.

Nystoriak, M., Bhatnagar, A. 'Cardiovascular Effects and Benefits of Exercise', *Frontiers in Cardiovascular Medicine*, vol. 5, no. 135, 2018.

Mandsager, K., Harb, S., Cremer, P., Phelan, D., Nissen, S., Jaber,

W. 'Association of Cardiorespiratory Fitness with Long-term Mortality Among Adults Undergoing Exercise Treadmill Testing', *JAMA Network Open*, vol. 1, no. 6, 2018.

Gill, J.M.R. 'Linking volume and intensity of physical activity to mortality', *Nat Med.*, vol. 26, 2020, pp. 1332–1334. https://doi. org/10.1038/s41591-020-1019-9.

Egan, B., Zierath, J.R. 'Exercise Metabolism and the Molecular Regulation of Skeletal Muscle Adaptation', *Cell Metabolism*, vol. 17, no. 2, 2013, pp. 162–184. doi: https://doi. org/10.1016/j.cmet.2012.12.012.

Ramos, J., Dalleck, L., Tjonna, A., Beetham, K., Coombes, J. 'The Impact of High-Intensity Interval Training Versus Moderate-Intensity Continuous Training on Vascular Function: a Systematic Review and Meta-Analysis', *Sports Medicine*, vol. 45, 2015, pp. 679–692.

Viana, R., Naves, J., Coswig, V., De Lira, C., Steele, J., Fisher, J., Gentil, P. 'Is interval training the magic bullet for fat loss? A systematic review and meta-analysis comparing moderate-intensity continuous training with high-intensity interval training (HIIT)', *British Journal of Sports Medicine*, vol. 53, no. 10, 2018.

Boudoulas, K., Borer, J., Boudoulas, H. 'Heart Rate, Life Expectancy and the Cardiovascular System: Therapeutic Considerations', *Cardiology*, vol. 132, no. 4, 2015, pp. 199–212.

Zhao, M., Veeranki, S., Magnussen, C., Xi, B. 'Recommended physical activity and all-cause and cause-specific mortality in US adults: Prospective cohort study', *British Medical Journal*, vol. 370, 2020.

Faulkner, J., Larkin, L., Claflin, D., Brooks, S. 'Age-related changes in the structure and function of skeletal muscles', *Clinical and Experimental Pharmacology and Physiology*, vol. 34, no. 11, 2007, pp. 1091–1096.

Srikanthan, P., Karlamangla, A. 'Muscle mass index as a predictor of longevity in older adults', *American Journal of Medicine*, vol. 127, no. 6, 2014, pp. 547–553.

Rantanen, T., Harris, T. et al. 'Muscle Strength and Body Mass

Index as Long-Term Predictors of Mortality in Initially Healthy Men', *Journals of Gerontology, Series A: Biological Sciences and Medical Sciences*, vol. 55, no. 3, 2000, pp. M168–M173.

Schuelke, M. et al. 'Myostatin Mutation Associated with Gross Muscle Hypertrophy in a Child', *New England Journal of Medicine*, vol. 350, 2004, pp. 2682–2688.

Walker, K., Kambadur, R., Sharma, M., Smith, H. 'Resistance Training Alters Plasma Myostatin but not IGF-1 in Healthy Men', *Medicine & Science in Sports & Exercise*, vol. 36, no. 5, 2004, pp. 787–793.

Nash, S., Liao, L., Harris, T., Freedman, N. 'Cigarette Smoking and Mortality in Adults Aged 70 Years and Older: Results From the NIH-AARP Cohort', *American Journal of Preventive Medicine*, vol. 52, no. 3, 2017, pp. 276–283.

Chapter 24: Mind Over Matter

Moseley, J. et al. 'A controlled trial of arthroscopic surgery for osteoarthritis of the knee', *New England Journal of Medicine*, vol. 347, 2002, pp. 81–88.

Guevarra, D. et al. 'Placebos without deception reduce self-report and neural measures of emotional distress', *Nature Communications*, vol. 11, no. 3785, 2020.

Kaptchuk, T. et al. 'Placebos without deception: A randomized controlledtrial in irritable bowel syndrome', *PLOS ONE*, vol. 5, no. 12, 2010.

Park, C., Pagnini, F., Langer, E. 'Glucose metabolism responds to perceived sugar intake more than actual sugar intake', *Sci Rep.*, 10: 15633, 2020. https://doi.org/10.1038/s41598-020-72501-w.

Westerhof, G., Miche, M. et al. 'The influence of subjective aging on health and longevity: A meta-analysis of longitudinal data', *Psychology and Aging*, vol. 29, no. 4, 2014, pp. 793–802.

John, A., Patel, U., Rusted, J., Richards, M., Gaysina, D. 'Affective

problems and decline in cognitive state in older adults: A systematic review and meta-analysis', *Psychological Medicine*, vol. 49,
no. 3, 2019, pp. 353–365.

Turnwald, B. et al. 'Learning one's genetic risk changes physiology
independent of actual genetic risk', *Nature Human Behaviour*,
vol. 3, 2019, pp. 48–56.

Kramer, C., Mehmood, S., Suen, R. 'Dog ownership and survival:
A systematic review and meta-analysis', *Circulation: Cardiovascular
Quality and Outcomes*, vol. 12, no. 10, 2019.

Pressman, S., Cohen, S. 'Use of social words in autobiographies and
longevity', *Psychosomatic Medicine*, vol. 69, no. 3, 2007, pp. 262–269.

Headey, B., Yong, J. 'Happiness and Longevity: Unhappy People Die
Young, Otherwise Happiness Probably Makes No Difference',
Social Indicators Research, vol. 142, no. 2, 2019, pp. 713–732.

Silk, J. et al. 'Strong and consistent social bonds enhance the longevity of female baboons', *Current Biology*, vol. 20, no. 15, 2010,
pp. 1359–1361.

Index